Dosages and Solutions:
A Programmed Approach
to Meds and Math
fifth edition

Dosages and Solutions:
A Programmed Approach
to Meds and Math
fifth edition

EMILY F. CORNETT, RN, PhD
Associate Professor
The University of Texas at Austin
School of Nursing
Austin, Texas

DOROTHY M. BLUME, RN, MSN
Associate Professor, Retired
The University of Texas at Austin
School of Nursing
Austin, Texas

 F. A. DAVIS COMPANY • Philadelphia

Printed in the United States of America

Last digit indicates print number: 10 9 8 7 6 5 4 3 2

NOTE: As new scientific information becomes available through basic and clinical research, recommended treatments and drug therapies undergo changes. The author(s) and publisher have done everything possible to make this book accurate, up-to-date, and in accord with accepted standards at the time of publication. The authors, editors, and publisher are not responsible for errors or omissions or for consequences from application of the book, and make no warranty, expressed or implied, in regard to the contents of the book. Any practice described in this book should be applied by the reader in accordance with professional standards of care used in regard to the unique circumstances that may apply in each situation. The reader is advised always to check product information (package inserts) for changes and new information regarding dose and contraindications before administering any drug. Caution is especially urged when using new or infrequently ordered drugs.

Library of Congress Cataloging-in-Publication Data

Cornett, Emily F., 1932–
　　Dosages and solutions: a programmed approach to meds and math /
　Emily F. Cornett, Dorothy M. Blume.—Ed. 5.
　　　p. cm.
　　Blume's name appears first on the 4th ed.
　　Includes bibliographical references and index.
　　ISBN 0-8036-1981-2 (softbound: alk. paper)
　　1. Drugs—Dosage—Problems, exercises, etc. 2. Solutions (Pharmacy)—Problems, exercises, etc. I. Blume, Dorothy M. II. Title.
　　[DNLM: 1. Drugs—administration & dosage. 2. Solutions—programmed instruction.　QV 18 C816d]
　RM145.B55　1991
　615′.14—dc20
　DLC
　for Library of Congress

91-9455
CIP

Medication Label Photographs and
Syringe Illustrations by David Fudell
Graphics Staff
The University of Texas at Austin
School of Nursing
Austin, Texas

Preface

Dosages and Solutions has been written primarily for nursing students. However, it also can be of value for in-service education programs, for refresher courses for inactive nurses, and as a desk reference for nurses and other health-care practitioners who administer medications wherever they are employed. An early introduction to classroom laboratory problems using sample drug labels and equipment is suggested for users of this book.

This book offers a practical approach to the preparation of drug dosages and solutions. Suggested methods of doing most drug dosage calculations have been reduced to two variations of using ratio and proportion. To the extent feasible, the content presented goes from simple to complex. However, examples have been selected to reflect realistic situations, therefore difficult problems sometimes are encountered in the examples of preparing drugs and solutions for administration.

The Arithmetic Basics section has been moved to the front of the book as requested by many users and other reviewers to allow the user a review of arithmetic skills before beginning drug calculations. Users whose math skills need no review can begin with Chapter 2 of the book.

Learning objectives have been added for each chapter. The information most often needed by practitioners has been placed on 3-inch by 5-inch cards on a perforated sheet of heavy paper at the back the book. These cards can be carried into the clinical setting and used as a reference for fluid and drug administration calculations.

Other additions include more pictures of actual drug labels and drug administration equipment, the use of military time, newer drugs such as human insulins, and precautions for giving medications to older adults. The official International System of Units (IU), or the French Système International d'Unités, metric measure abbreviations have been used throughout the book.

In Appendix C, answers to all problems are followed by the page number in the text to which the user can refer if difficulty is encountered when working the problem. Thus the user has quick access not just to the correct answer but to the content needed to be mastered to yield that answer.

At the suggestion of college of pharmacy faculty and practicing pharmacists, the Apothecaries' system has been retained. Although seldom used, the preparation of oral and topical solutions from powders, crystals, tablets, or stronger solutions has been retained because students better understand the strength of other drug solutions once they study this section.

Outdated drugs and equipment have been deleted. Young's, Fried's, and Clark's Rules for pediatric dosages have been moved to Appendix B for reference, if needed. Children's dosage problems have been deleted from all but the intravenous administration sections and the chapter on pediatric doses.

Medication administration records and medication cards have not been included as was suggested by a few reviewers. Our opinion is that because the forms and formats differ considerably among health-care agencies, it would not be useful to have the learner practice on forms they never see. Also, in many agencies, written records are not used since medications records are kept on computers.

We wish to express our sincere appreciation to students and to faculty members in schools of nursing whose comments and helpful suggestions have guided this revision. We especially want to thank those nurses and pharmacists in local hospitals and teaching institutions for their contributions to this edition.

Emily F. Cornett, RN, PhD
Dorothy M. Blume, RN, MSN

Consultants

Deborah J. Borelli, RN
St. Petersburg Junior College
St. Petersburg, Florida

Jill W. Brown, RN
Florida Atlantic University
Boca Raton, Florida

Karon Overmeyer, RN
Professor
Broward Community College
Department of Nursing Technology
Davie, Florida

Gretchen Vancura, RN
Harper College
Palatine, Illinois

Betty Wade, RN
Texas Woman's University
College of Nursing
Dallas, Texas

Contents

CHAPTER 1

Arithmetic Basics

Some individuals prefer to have a basic arithmetic review prior to beginning the calculations of drug dosages. This chapter provides that review and practice problems in areas in which users may find that they need additional practice. Users who do not need an arithmetic review can proceed to Chapter 2, Overview, which presents the systems of measurement and methods of calculation used in preparing drug dosages and solutions.

OBJECTIVES

At the end of this chapter, the student should be able to:
- Add, subtract, multiply, and divide common fractions
- Add, subtract, multiply, and divide decimal fractions
- Make common and decimal fractions, percent, and ratio conversions
- Understand the components and relationships of ratios and proportions
- Determine the unknown mean or extreme in a proportion
- Make Celsius and Fahrenheit degree conversions
- Make Roman and Arabic numeral conversions
- Make standard and military time conversions

PART 1 • Arithmetic Pretest

Answers can be found in Appendix C, pp. 233–235.

Which is larger:

1. $\frac{1}{150}$ or $\frac{1}{200}$?

2. $\frac{3}{7}$ or $\frac{3}{8}$?

3. $\frac{100}{1}$ or $\frac{3}{2}$?

4. 0.006 or 0.03?

5. 1:20 or 1:2?

6. $\frac{1}{10}\%$ or $\frac{1}{5}\%$?

7. $\frac{1}{100}$ or $\frac{2}{100}$?

8. 0.030 or 0.04?

9. 0.066 or 0.06?

Complete the following:

10. $\frac{300}{150} + \frac{4}{3} =$

11. $\frac{3}{2} + \frac{4}{3} =$

12. $1\frac{1}{4} + \frac{1}{6} =$

13. $\frac{1}{1000} + 2\frac{1}{2} =$

14. $\frac{2}{7} + \frac{2}{3} =$

15. $\frac{1}{100} + \frac{1}{100} =$

16. $1\frac{1}{2} + \frac{3}{4} =$

17. $\frac{1}{2} + \frac{1}{3} + 1\frac{1}{4} =$

18. $\frac{1}{4}\% + \frac{1}{3}\% =$

19. $0.04 + 0.033 =$

20. $1:5 + 4:6 =$

21. $4\frac{1}{2} - 3 =$

22. $\frac{1}{100} - \frac{1}{150} =$

23. $\frac{4}{3} - \frac{7}{6} =$

24. $1\frac{1}{2} - 1\frac{1}{3} =$

25. $0.66 - 0.06 =$

26. $\frac{1}{1000} \times 1 =$

27. $0.03 \times 2 =$

28. $\frac{100}{1} \times 5 =$

29. $\frac{2}{3} \times \frac{1}{2} =$

30. $1\frac{1}{2} \times \frac{1}{3} =$

31. $1\frac{1}{2} \div \frac{1}{3} =$

32. $\frac{300}{150} \div 2 =$

33. $\frac{3}{4} \div \frac{2}{3} =$

34. $1.5 \div 0.1 =$

35. $0.5 \div \frac{3}{4} =$

36. $\dfrac{\frac{1}{3}}{\frac{1}{2}} =$

37. $\dfrac{1\frac{1}{2}}{2} =$

Change to decimal fractions:

38. $\frac{1}{10} =$

39. $2\% =$

40. $\frac{15}{1} =$

41. $2:50 =$

Change to ratios:

42. $0.03 =$

43. $1 =$

44. $75\% =$

45. $\frac{1}{1000} =$

46. $0.5\% =$

47. $0.125\% =$

Change to percent:

48. $\frac{1}{300} =$

49. $\frac{1}{2} =$

50. $1:1000 =$

51. $0.75 =$

52. $2\frac{1}{2} =$

Solve for x, the unknown value:

53. $400:1 = 1000:x$

54. $80:16 = 100:x$

55. $15:1000 = x:100$

56. $\dfrac{1}{10,000} : \dfrac{1}{8000} = x:4000$

57. $100:1000 = \frac{1}{4}:x$

Round off to the nearest 10th:

58. $0.33 =$

59. $0.6\frac{2}{3} =$

Round off to the nearest 100th:

60. $0.666\frac{2}{3} =$

61. $0.3\frac{1}{3} =$

Write these Roman numerals in Arabic numbers:

62. IX =

63. vi =

64. XC =

65. XII =

66. LX =

Write these Arabic numbers in Roman numerals:

67. 4 =

68. 2000 =

69. 6 =

70. 15 =

71. 100 =

Change to degrees (°) C:

72. 97°F =

73. −40°F =

74. 110°F =

75. 65°F =

76. 105°F =

Change to degrees (°) F:

77. 10°C =

78. 40°C =

79. −10°C =

80. 32°C =

81. 37°C =

Change standard time to military time:

82. 12:30 AM =

83. 4:20 PM =

84. 10:15 AM =

85. 7:30 AM =

86. 9:00 PM =

Change military time to standard time:

87. 2400 =

88. 0015 =

89. 2100 =

90. 1530 =

91. 0900 =

92. 0730 =

PART 2 • Arithmetic Review

COMMON FRACTIONS

Definitions

A **proper fraction** is one in which the numerator is less than the denominator. The numerator is the top number and the denominator is the bottom number of the fraction.
  Examples:

$$\tfrac{1}{2} \quad \tfrac{2}{3} \quad \tfrac{1}{200} \quad \tfrac{150}{200}$$
$$\tfrac{3}{4} \quad \tfrac{5}{6} \quad \tfrac{1}{1000} \quad \tfrac{3}{1000}$$

An **improper fraction** is one in which the numerator is equal to, or greater than, the denominator.
  Examples:

$$\tfrac{2}{2} \quad \tfrac{4}{3} \quad \tfrac{3000}{2000} \quad \tfrac{5}{4}$$
$$\tfrac{7}{5} \quad \tfrac{300}{150} \quad \tfrac{150}{150} \quad \tfrac{200}{150}$$

A **whole number** has an unexpressed denominator of one (1).
  Examples:

$$4 = \tfrac{4}{1} \quad 1000 = \tfrac{1000}{1} \quad 500 = \tfrac{500}{1}$$
$$1 = \tfrac{1}{1} \quad 60 = \tfrac{60}{1} \quad 2 = \tfrac{2}{1}$$

A **mixed number** is a whole number plus a fraction.
  Examples:

$$1\tfrac{1}{3} \quad 10\tfrac{2}{3} \quad 1\tfrac{1}{2} \quad 40\tfrac{1}{4}$$
$$2\tfrac{1}{2} \quad 25\tfrac{7}{8} \quad 7\tfrac{1}{2} \quad 5\tfrac{1}{2}$$

A **complex fraction** is one in which the numerator, denominator, or both, are fractions.
  Examples:

$$\frac{1\tfrac{1}{2}}{2} \quad \frac{\tfrac{1}{1000}}{1} \quad \frac{\tfrac{1}{3}}{\tfrac{1}{2}} \quad \frac{1}{\tfrac{1}{100}}$$

Changing Common Fractions

An **improper fraction** can be changed to a **whole or a mixed number** by dividing the numerator by the denominator.
  Examples:

$$\tfrac{7}{5} = 7 \div 5 = 1\tfrac{2}{7}$$
$$\tfrac{150}{25} = 150 \div 25 = 6$$
$$\tfrac{1000}{1000} = 1000 \div 1000 = 1$$
$$\tfrac{300}{150} = 300 \div 150 = 2$$

A **mixed number** can be changed to an **improper fraction** by multiplying the whole number by the denominator, adding the numerator, and placing the sum over the denominator.

Examples:

$$1\frac{1}{3} = \frac{3 \times 1 + 1}{3} = \frac{4}{3}$$

$$3\frac{3}{4} = \frac{3 \times 4 + 3}{4} = \frac{15}{4}$$

$$7\frac{1}{2} = \frac{7 \times 2 + 1}{2} = \frac{15}{2}$$

$$33\frac{1}{3} = \frac{33 \times 3 + 1}{3} = \frac{100}{3}$$

To **simplify a complex fraction,** divide the numerator by the denominator after reducing either or both, as needed, to a simpler fraction.
Examples:

$$\frac{7\frac{1}{2}}{5} = \frac{15/2}{5} = \frac{15}{2} \div \frac{5}{1} = \frac{15}{2} \times \frac{1}{5} = \frac{15}{10} = 1\frac{1}{2}$$

$$\frac{1\frac{1}{2}}{2} = \frac{3/2}{2} = \frac{3}{2} \div \frac{2}{1} = \frac{3}{2} \times \frac{1}{2} = \frac{3}{4}$$

Comparing Sizes of Common Fractions

Comparing sizes of common fractions often is very important for those administering medications.

If the **numerators are the same,** the fraction with the smaller denominator represents the larger value.
Examples:

½ is larger than ¼
$\frac{1}{150}$ is larger than $\frac{1}{300}$

If the **denominators are the same,** the fraction with the larger numerator represents the larger value.
Examples:

$\frac{2}{300}$ is larger than $\frac{1}{300}$
¾ is larger than ¼

Fractions with different denominators can be compared by changing both denominators to the same denominator.
Examples:

$\frac{1}{150}$ ($\frac{2}{300}$) is larger than $\frac{1}{300}$
⅙ ($\frac{5}{30}$) is smaller than ⅕ ($\frac{6}{30}$)

Adding Common Fractions

To add common fractions, change fractions to equivalent fractions with the least common denominator, add the numerators, and write this sum over the common denominator. A least common denominator is the smallest number into which all denominators can be divided evenly.

Examples of **proper fractions**:

$$\tfrac{1}{200} + \tfrac{1}{100} = \tfrac{1}{200} + \tfrac{2}{200} = \tfrac{3}{200}$$

$$\tfrac{1}{300} + \tfrac{1}{150} + \tfrac{1}{10} = \tfrac{1}{300} + \tfrac{2}{300} + \tfrac{30}{300} = \tfrac{33}{300} = \tfrac{11}{100}$$

Examples of **improper fractions**:

$$\tfrac{1}{1} + \tfrac{4}{3} + \tfrac{9}{7} = \tfrac{21}{21} + \tfrac{28}{21} + \tfrac{27}{21} = \tfrac{76}{21} = 3\tfrac{13}{21}$$

$$\tfrac{2}{1} + \tfrac{7}{4} + \tfrac{10}{8} = \tfrac{16}{8} + \tfrac{14}{8} + \tfrac{10}{8} = \tfrac{40}{8} = 5$$

Examples of **mixed numbers**:

$$1\tfrac{1}{3} + 2\tfrac{1}{2} = \tfrac{4}{3} + \tfrac{5}{2} = \tfrac{8}{6} + \tfrac{15}{6} = \tfrac{23}{6} = 3\tfrac{5}{6}$$

$$1\tfrac{3}{4} + 1\tfrac{1}{2} = \tfrac{7}{4} + \tfrac{3}{2} = \tfrac{7}{4} + \tfrac{6}{4} = \tfrac{13}{4} = 3\tfrac{1}{4}$$

Examples of **whole and mixed numbers and fractions**:

$$1\tfrac{1}{2} + \tfrac{3}{4} = \tfrac{3}{2} + \tfrac{3}{4} = \tfrac{6}{4} + \tfrac{3}{4} = \tfrac{9}{4} = 2\tfrac{1}{4}$$

$$2 + \tfrac{1}{2} = \tfrac{2}{1} + \tfrac{1}{2} = \tfrac{4}{2} + \tfrac{1}{2} = \tfrac{5}{2} = 2\tfrac{1}{2}$$

Subtracting Common Fractions

To **subtract** common fractions, again reduce to equivalent fractions with the least common denominator, subtract the numerator after the minus sign from the numerator before the minus sign, and place the remainder over the common denominator.

Examples of **proper fractions**:

$$\tfrac{1}{2} - \tfrac{1}{3} = \tfrac{3}{6} - \tfrac{2}{6} = \tfrac{1}{6}$$

$$\tfrac{1}{150} - \tfrac{1}{300} = \tfrac{2}{300} - \tfrac{1}{300} = \tfrac{1}{300}$$

Examples of **improper fractions**:

$$\tfrac{3}{2} - \tfrac{5}{4} = \tfrac{6}{4} - \tfrac{5}{4} = \tfrac{1}{4}$$

$$\tfrac{300}{150} - \tfrac{300}{200} = \tfrac{1200}{600} - \tfrac{900}{600} = \tfrac{300}{600} = \tfrac{1}{2}$$

Examples of **mixed numbers**:

$$1\tfrac{1}{3} - 1\tfrac{1}{4} = \tfrac{4}{3} - \tfrac{5}{4} = \tfrac{16}{12} - \tfrac{15}{12} = \tfrac{1}{12}$$

$$4\tfrac{3}{4} - 2\tfrac{1}{2} = 4\tfrac{3}{4} - 2\tfrac{2}{4} = 2\tfrac{1}{4}$$

Examples of **whole and mixed numbers and fractions**:

$$5 - 2\tfrac{1}{2} = \tfrac{5}{1} - \tfrac{5}{2} = \tfrac{10}{2} - \tfrac{5}{2} = \tfrac{5}{2} = 2\tfrac{1}{2}$$

$$1\tfrac{1}{2} - \tfrac{1}{4} = \tfrac{3}{2} - \tfrac{1}{4} = \tfrac{6}{4} - \tfrac{1}{4} = \tfrac{5}{4} = 1\tfrac{1}{4}$$

Multiplying Common Fractions

To **multiply common fractions,** multiply the numerators together and the denominators together, then reduce the resulting fraction to its lowest terms.

Examples of **proper fractions**:

$$\tfrac{2}{3} \times \tfrac{3}{4} = \tfrac{6}{12} = \tfrac{1}{2}$$

$$\tfrac{1}{100} \times \tfrac{1}{2} = \tfrac{1}{200}$$

Examples of **improper fractions**:

$$2/1 \times 3/2 = 6/2 = 3$$

$$300/150 \times 1/1 = 300/150 = 2$$

Examples of **mixed numbers**:

$$1\tfrac{1}{3} \times 2\tfrac{1}{2} = 4/3 \times 5/2 = 20/6 = 3\tfrac{2}{6} = 3\tfrac{1}{3}$$

$$1/1000 \times 1/2 = 1000/2 = 500$$

Examples of **whole and mixed numbers by fractions**:

$$2 \times 1/100 = 2/1 \times 1/100 = 2/100 = 1/50$$

$$1\tfrac{1}{2} \times 1/1000 = 3/2 \times 1/1000 = 3/2000$$

Dividing Common Fractions

To **divide common fractions,** invert the divisor and multiply.
  Examples of **proper fractions**:

$$2/3 \div 3/4 = 2/3 \times 4/3 = 8/9$$

$$1/100 \div 1/500 = 1/100 \times 500/1 = 500/100 = 5$$

Examples of **improper fractions**:

$$3/2 \div 2/1 = 3/2 \times 1/2 = 3/4$$

$$300/150 \div 2/1 = 300/150 \times 1/2 = 300/300 = 1$$

Examples of **mixed numbers**:

$$1\tfrac{1}{2} \div 2\tfrac{1}{3} = 3/2 \div 7/3 = 3/2 \times 3/7 = 9/14$$

$$1\tfrac{1}{100} \div 2\tfrac{1}{4} = 101/100 \div 5/4 = 101/100 \times 4/5 = 404/500 = 101/125$$

Examples of **whole and mixed numbers by fractions**:

$$1\tfrac{1}{2} \div 3/4 = 3/2 \div 3/4 = 3/2 \times 4/3 = 12/6 = 2$$

$$500 \div 1/1000 = 500/1 \div 1/1000 = 500/1 \times 1000/1 = 500,000/1 = 500,000$$

DECIMAL FRACTIONS
Definition

A **decimal fraction** is a fraction whose denominator is any power of 10 and which may
be expressed in decimal form.

Changing Decimal Fractions to and from Common Fractions

Changing **common fractions to decimal fractions** is done by dividing the numerator
by the denominator.

Examples:

$$\frac{0.5}{\tfrac{1}{2} = 2)\,1.0} \qquad\qquad 7\tfrac{1}{2} = {}^{15}\!/_2 = \frac{7.5}{2)\,15.0}$$

$$\frac{0.005}{\tfrac{1}{200} = 200)\,1.000} \qquad\qquad {}^{1000}\!/_2 = \frac{500}{2)\,1000.0}$$

Changing **decimal fractions to common fractions** is done more easily but great care should be taken in determining the correct denominator.

Examples:

0.1	$= {}^1\!/_{10}$	or one-tenth
0.01	$= {}^1\!/_{100}$	or one-hundredth
0.001	$= {}^1\!/_{1000}$	or one-thousandth
0.0001	$= {}^1\!/_{10,000}$	or one ten-thousandth
7.5	$= {}^{75}\!/_{10}$	
0.33	$= {}^{33}\!/_{100}$	
0.667	$= {}^{667}\!/_{1000}$	
0.0003	$= {}^3\!/_{10,000}$	

Comparing Sizes of Decimal Fractions

Comparing the sizes of decimal fractions often is very important for those administering medications.

The **higher the whole number** preceding the decimal point, the higher the value of the decimal number.

Examples:

> 4.25 is of greater value than 3.75
> 17.5 is of greater value than 16.9

If there are **no whole numbers** to the left of the decimal point or the whole numbers are the same, the numerical value to the right of the decimal point will determine which number has the greater value:

First, the fraction with the higher number at the 10th position has the greater value.

Examples:

> 2.25 is of greater value than 2.1
> 0.3 is of greater value than 0.25
> 0.7 is of greater value than 0.667

Second, if the numbers at the 10th position are the same, then the higher number at the 100th position has the greater value.

Examples:

> 7.75 is of greater value than 7.7
> 0.67 is of greater value than 0.665
> 0.05 is of greater value than 0.045

Third, if the numbers at the 100th position are the same, then the higher number at the 1000th position has the greater value.

Examples:

> 0.333 is of greater value than 0.33
> 0.005 is of greater value than 0.004
> 1.015 is of greater value than 1.0125

When there is no whole number in a decimal fraction, a zero is placed in front of the decimal point to indicate that no whole number has been omitted.

Rounding Off Decimal Fractions

To **round decimal fractions to the nearest 10th,** drop numbers of four or less at the 100th position. When the number at the 100th position is five or more, add one 10th.
Examples:

$$1.33 \text{ rounds to } 1.3$$
$$1.66 \text{ rounds to } 1.7$$
$$0.05 \text{ rounds to } 0.1$$
$$0.025 \text{ rounds to } 0.0$$
$$0.075 \text{ rounds to } 0.1$$

To **round decimal fractions to the nearest 100th,** drop numbers of four or less at the 1000th position. When the number at the 1000th position is five or more, add one 100th.
Examples:

$$1.333 \text{ rounds to } 1.33$$
$$1.666 \text{ rounds to } 1.67$$
$$0.005 \text{ rounds to } 0.01$$
$$0.025 \text{ rounds to } 0.03$$
$$0.033 \text{ rounds to } 0.03$$

Adding and Subtracting Decimal Fractions

To **add or subtract decimal fractions,** place the decimal points in vertical alignment, add zeros to carry all fractions to the same position, and add or subtract from right to left.
Examples of **adding**:

$$0.0004 + 0.006 = \begin{array}{r} 0.0004 \\ + 0.0060 \\ \hline 0.0064 \end{array}$$

$$3.333 + 0.05 = \begin{array}{r} 3.333 \\ + 0.050 \\ \hline 3.383 \end{array}$$

Examples of **subtracting**:

$$0.06 - 0.004 = \begin{array}{r} 0.060 \\ - 0.004 \\ \hline 0.056 \end{array}$$

$$7.75 - 5.025 = \begin{array}{r} 7.750 \\ - 5.025 \\ \hline 2.725 \end{array}$$

Multiplying Decimal Fractions

To **multiply decimal fractions,** first multiply as with whole numbers. Second, in the product, count off from right to left as many decimal places as there are in both the multiplicand and the multiplier.

Examples:

$$\begin{array}{r} \text{(Multiplicand)} \quad \text{(Multiplier)} \\ 1.25 \times 0.75 \quad = \quad 1.25 \\ \times\, 0.75 \\ \hline 625 \\ 875 \\ \hline 0.9375 \ \text{(Product)} \end{array}$$

$$\begin{array}{r} 1.5 \times 0.67 \quad = \quad 1.50 \\ 0.67 \\ \hline 1050 \\ 900 \\ \hline 1.0050 \end{array}$$

Dividing Decimal Fractions

To **divide decimal fractions,** divide as with whole numbers **after** converting the divisor to a whole number by moving the decimal point to the far right and **after** moving the decimal point in the dividend the same number of places to the right, adding zeros as necessary.

Examples:

$$\begin{array}{r} \text{(Dividend)} \quad \text{(Divisor)} \qquad\qquad 1.5 \ \text{(Quotient)} \\ 1.125 \div 0.75 \quad = \quad 0.75\overline{)1.125} \\ 75 \\ \hline 375 \\ 375 \\ \hline 000 \end{array}$$

$$\begin{array}{r} \qquad\qquad\qquad\qquad 20. \\ 0.6 \div 0.03 \quad = \quad 0.03\overline{)0.60} \\ 60 \\ \hline 000 \end{array}$$

PERCENTAGE

Definition

A **percent** is a part of 100 equal parts. It is a fraction with an implied denominator of 100.

Examples:

$$5\% = {}^{5}\!/_{100} \qquad\qquad 2.5\% = {}^{2.5}\!/_{100}$$
$$0.1\% = {}^{0.1}\!/_{100} \qquad\qquad 0.001\% = {}^{0.001}\!/_{100}$$

Changing Percents to and from Fractions

To **change percent to a common fraction,** write the numerical percent value as the numerator and replace the percent sign (%) with 100 as the denominator of the fraction.

Examples:

$$5\% = {}^5\!/_{100} = {}^1\!/_{20}$$

$$\frac{1}{10}\% = \frac{{}^1\!/_{10}}{100} = {}^1\!/_{10} \div {}^{100}\!/_1 = {}^1\!/_{10} \times {}^1\!/_{100} = {}^1\!/_{1000}$$

$$0.2\% = \frac{{}^2\!/_{10}}{100} = {}^2\!/_{10} \div {}^{100}\!/_1 = {}^2\!/_{10} \times {}^1\!/_{100} = {}^2\!/_{1000} = {}^1\!/_{500}$$

To **change common fractions to percent,** divide the numerator by the denominator and multiply the quotient by 100, which is the same as moving the decimal point two places to the right. Then add the percent sign.

Examples:

$$\frac{1}{8} = 8\overline{)1.000}^{\,0.125} = 0.125 \times 100 = 12.5\%$$

$$\begin{array}{r} 8 \\ \hline 20 \\ 16 \\ \hline 40 \\ 40 \\ \hline 00 \end{array}$$

$$\frac{3}{5} = 5\overline{)3.0}^{\,0.6} = 0.6 \times 100 = 60\%$$

$$\begin{array}{r} 30 \\ \hline 00 \end{array}$$

$$\frac{1}{1000} = 1000\overline{)1.000}^{\,0.001} = 0.001 \times 100 = 0.1\%$$

To **change percent to decimal fractions,** drop the percent sign and divide by 100, which is the same as moving the decimal point two places to the left.

Examples:

$$12.5\% = 0.125 \qquad\qquad 50\% = 0.50$$

$$100\overline{)12.500}^{\,0.125} \qquad\qquad \begin{array}{l} 0.75\% = 0.0075 \\ 0.7\% = 0.007 \\ 60\% = 0.6 \\ 0.1\% = 0.001 \\ 0.001\% = 0.00001 \end{array}$$

$$\begin{array}{r} 100 \\ \hline 250 \\ 200 \\ \hline 500 \\ 500 \\ \hline 000 \end{array}$$

To **change a decimal fraction to percent,** multiply the decimal fraction by 100, which is the same as moving the decimal point two places to the right. Then add the percent sign.

Examples:

$$0.05 = 5\% \qquad\qquad \begin{array}{l} 1.05 = 105\% \\ 0.25 = 25\% \\ 0.001 = 0.1\% \\ 0.2 = 20\% \\ 0.9 = 90\% \end{array}$$

$$\begin{array}{r} 0.05 \\ \times\ \ 100 \\ \hline 005.00 \end{array}$$

RATIO AND PROPORTION

Definitions

A **ratio** is the same as a fraction. The ratio 1:20 means that in every 20 total parts of a solution there is one part of powdered or crystal drug or other substance (called a solute) in 20 equivalent measures of a solution (called a solvent). It is like saying that in a 1:20 solution of sugar there is one part sugar (solute) in 20 equal measure parts of water (solvent).

Examples:

$$1:20 \quad 2:400 \quad 1:1000$$
$$0.1:100 \quad 5:100 \quad 0.9:100$$

A **proportion** consists of two ratios or fractions that are of equal value. The ratio 1:20 is the same as the ratio 5:100. These two ratios have the same relative values, or they are said to be "in proportion." Therefore, 1:20 = 5:100.

Examples:

$$1:4 = 2:8 \qquad 1:400 = 2:800$$
$$1:4 = 400:1600 \qquad 1:500 = 0.5:250$$
$$1:2 = 1000:2000 \qquad 100:16 = 200:32$$

The first and last terms of a proportion are called the **extremes**. The second and third terms are called the **means**. If the ratios in the proportion are equal in value, **the product of two means will equal the product of the two extremes**.

Examples:

<pre>
        Means
      ┌──────┐
   25 : 100 = 50 : 200   100 × 50 = 5000 (Means)
   └──────────────┘
      Extremes   25 × 200 = 5000 (Extremes)

        Means
       ┌─────┐
   0.1 : 100 = 0.5 : 500   100 × 0.5 = 50 (Means)
   └───────────────┘
       Extremes   0.1 × 500 = 50 (Extremes)
</pre>

Ratio and Proportion Equations

Any one number of a ratio and proportion equation may be unknown and is represented in the equation by an x.

An **unknown mean** indicates that either the second or third term of a proportion is unknown and is, therefore, indicated by an x.

Examples:

$$25:100 = x:200$$
$$0.1:x = 0.5:500$$

An **unknown extreme** indicates that either the first or fourth term of a proportion is unknown and is indicated by an x.

Examples:

$$x:100 = 50:200$$
$$500:0.5 = 100:x$$

Determining the Value of x

When any three of the four terms of a proportion are known, the unknown fourth term can be calculated.

An **unknown mean** is found by dividing the product of the two known extremes by the one known mean. In other words, after multiplying the two means and the two extremes, divide both sides of the resulting equation by the number preceding x, the unknown mean.

Examples:

$$4:20 = x:25$$
$$20x = 100$$
$$1x\,(20x \div 20) = 5\,(100 \div 20)$$
$$x = 5$$

$$1:500 = x:400$$
$$500x = 400$$
$$x = {}^{400}\!/_{500}$$
$$x = 0.8$$

$$0.5:200 = x:300$$
$$200x = 150$$
$$x = 0.75$$

$${}^1\!/_{100}:x = {}^1\!/_{150}:1$$
$${}^1\!/_{150}x = {}^1\!/_{100}$$
$$x = {}^1\!/_{100} \div {}^1\!/_{150}$$
$$x = {}^1\!/_{100} \times {}^{150}\!/_{1}$$
$$x = {}^{150}\!/_{100}$$
$$x = 1.5$$

An **unknown extreme** is found by dividing the product of the two known means by the one known extreme. In other words, after multiplying the two means and the two extremes, divide both sides of the resulting equation by the number preceding x, the unknown extreme.

Examples:

$$x:20 = 5:25$$
$$25x = 100$$
$$1x\,(25x \div 25) = 4\,(100 \div 25)$$
$$x = 4$$

$$4:20 = 5:x$$
$$4x = 100$$
$$x = {}^{100}\!/_{4}$$
$$x = 25$$

$$1:10,000 = 0.005:x$$
$$x = 50$$

$$x:{}^1\!/_{1000} = 1:{}^1\!/_{5000}$$
$${}^1\!/_{5000}x = {}^1\!/_{1000}$$
$$x = {}^1\!/_{1000} \div {}^1\!/_{5000}$$
$$x = {}^1\!/_{1000} \times {}^{5000}\!/_{1}$$
$$x = {}^{5000}\!/_{1000}$$
$$x = 5$$

$$x : 0.0025 = 1 : 0.005$$
$$0.005x = 0.0025$$
$$0.005x \div 0.005 = 0.0025 \div 0.005$$
$$x = 0.5$$

Changing Ratios to and from Fractions

To **change a common fraction to a ratio,** the numerator becomes the first term of the ratio and the denominator becomes the second term of the ratio.

    Examples:

$$\tfrac{1}{2} = 1:2$$
$$\tfrac{7}{5} = 7:5$$
$$1\tfrac{1}{3} = \tfrac{4}{3} = 4:3$$
$$\frac{1\tfrac{1}{2}}{2} = \frac{3}{2} \div \frac{2}{1} = \frac{3}{2} \times \frac{1}{2} = \frac{3}{4} = 3:4$$

To **change a ratio to a common fraction,** place the first term of the ratio as the numerator over the second term of the ratio as the denominator.

    Examples:

$$1:10{,}000 = \tfrac{1}{10{,}000}$$

$$64:3 = \tfrac{64}{3} = 21\tfrac{1}{3}$$

$$16:0.03 = \tfrac{16}{0.03} = \tfrac{1600}{3} = 532\tfrac{1}{3}$$

$$1:0.75 = \frac{1}{\tfrac{3}{4}} = \frac{1}{1} \div \frac{3}{4} = \frac{1}{1} \times \frac{4}{3} = \frac{4}{3} = 1\tfrac{1}{3}$$

To **change a decimal fraction to a ratio,** place the numerical value of the decimal fraction as the numerator over the denominator of the decimal fraction, which will be 10 or a multiple of 10.

    Examples:

$$0.1 = \tfrac{1}{10} = 1:10$$
$$0.05 = \tfrac{5}{100} = \tfrac{1}{20} = 1:20$$
$$0.001 = \tfrac{1}{1000} = 1:1000$$
$$0.66 = \tfrac{66}{100} = \tfrac{33}{50} = 33:50$$
$$0.333 = \tfrac{333}{1000} = 333:1000$$
$$1.25 = \tfrac{125}{100} = \tfrac{125}{100} = \tfrac{5}{4} = 5:4$$

To **change a ratio to a decimal fraction,** divide the first term of the ratio by the second term of the ratio.

    Examples:

$$5:100 = 0.05 \qquad\qquad 0.01:50 = 0.0002$$
$$1:1000 = 0.001$$

$$
\begin{array}{r}
0.05 \\
100\overline{)\,5.00} \\
500 \\
\hline
000
\end{array}
\qquad
\begin{array}{l}
2.25:100 = 0.0225 \\
1:100 = 0.01 \\
15:0.4 = 37.5 \\
1:10{,}000 = 0.0001
\end{array}
$$

To **change a percent to a ratio,** the numerical value becomes the first term of the ratio and the second term is always 100.

Examples:

$$0.9\% = 0.9:100 \qquad 0.001\% = 0.001:100$$
$$5\% = 5:100 \qquad 2\frac{1}{2}\% = 2.5:100$$
$$0.5\% = 0.5:100 \qquad 100\% = 100:100$$

To **change a ratio to a percent,** change the ratio to a common fraction, multiply by 100, and add the percent sign (%) to the answer.

Examples:

$$1:5 = \frac{1}{5} \times \frac{100}{1} = 20\%$$

$$0.4:100 = \frac{\frac{4}{10}}{100} \times \frac{100}{1} = \frac{4}{10} = 0.4\%$$

$$1:1000 = \frac{1}{1000} \times \frac{100}{1} = \frac{100}{1000} = \frac{1}{10} = 0.1\%$$

$$1:8 = \frac{1}{8} \times \frac{100}{1} = 12.5\%$$

CELSIUS-FAHRENHEIT CONVERSIONS

Thermal Scales

There are two thermal scales used in the United States—the degrees of Celsius (°C) and the degrees of Fahrenheit (°F). Most other countries use only the Celsius scale. At sea level, on the Celsius scale freezing is 0° and boiling is 100°, and on the Fahrenheit scale freezing is 32° and boiling is 212°, as shown in Figure 1–1.

Formulas for Converting Between Scales

To **convert from Fahrenheit to Celsius,** first subtract 32° from the °F, then multiply by $\frac{5}{9}$.

FORMULA: $°C = (°F - 32)\frac{5}{9}$

Examples:

212°F = ?°C $\qquad\qquad$ 60°F = ?°C
$°C = (212 - 32)\frac{5}{9}$ $\qquad$ $°C = (60 - 32)\frac{5}{9}$
$°C = 180 \times \frac{5}{9}$ $\qquad\quad$ $°C = 28 \times \frac{5}{9}$
$°C = 100°$ $\qquad\qquad\quad$ $°C = 15.6°$

32°F = ?°C $\qquad\qquad$ 98°F = ?°C
$°C = (32 - 32)\frac{5}{9}$ $\qquad$ $°C = (98 - 32)\frac{5}{9}$
$°C = 0 \times \frac{5}{9}$ $\qquad\quad$ $°C = 66 \times \frac{5}{9}$
$°C = 0°$ $\qquad\qquad\quad$ $°C = 36.67°$

To **convert Celsius to Fahrenheit,** first multiply the number of °C by $\frac{9}{5}$, then add 32°.

FORMULA: $°F = (°C \times \frac{9}{5}) + 32$

Examples:

100°C = ?°F $\qquad\qquad$ 0°C = ?°F
$°F = (100 \times \frac{9}{5}) + 32$ $\qquad$ $°F = (0 \times \frac{9}{5}) + 32$
$°F = 180 + 32$ $\qquad\qquad$ $°F = 0 + 32$
$°F = 212°$ $\qquad\qquad\quad$ $°F = 32°$

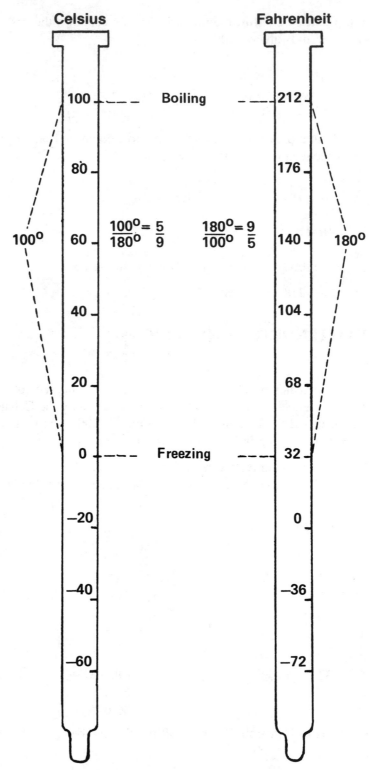

FIGURE 1–1 • Celsius and Fahrenheit thermometers.

$$40°C = ?°F \qquad\qquad 25°C = ?°F$$
$$°F = (40 \times \tfrac{9}{5}) + 32 \qquad °F = (25 \times \tfrac{9}{5}) + 32$$
$$°F = 72 + 32 \qquad\qquad °F = 45 + 32$$
$$°F = 104° \qquad\qquad °F = 77°$$

ROMAN AND ARABIC NUMERALS

Currently there are two systems of counting: Arabic numbers and Roman numerals. The Arabic system is used in the ordering and calculations of medication dosages. The Arabic numerals, or digits, are 1, 2, 3, 4, 5, 6, 7, 8, 9, and 0. They can be used with whole numbers, common fractions, decimal fractions, percentages, and ratios and proportions. This system is used with both metric and household measures. The decimal place values of Arabic numbers are shown in Table 1–1.

TABLE 1–1 • **Place Values of Arabic Numbers**		
Whole Numbers		*Decimal Fractions*
Millions	1,000,000	
Hundred thousands	100,000	
Ten thousands	10,000	
Thousands	1000	
Hundreds	100	
Tens	10	
Units	1	
No value	0.0	No value
	0.1	Tenths
	0.01	Hundredths
	0.001	Thousandths
	0.0001	Ten thousandths
	0.00001	Hundred thousandths
	0.000001	Millionths

Sometimes Roman numerals are used with the apothecaries' system to prescribe or calculate drug dosages. Seven capital letters may be used to express Roman numerals.

ROMAN NUMERALS	ARABIC NUMBERS
I	1
V	5
X	10
L	50
C	100
D	500
M	1000

Frequently lower case numerals are used to prescribe the amount of drugs or solutions, especially small amounts.

ROMAN NUMERALS	ARABIC NUMBERS
i or ï	1
v or $\bar{v}$	5
x or $\bar{x}$	10

A combination of Roman numerals are used to indicate other numbers. When a numeral of lesser value precedes a numeral of greater value, subtract the one of lesser value from the one of greater value. Only one numeral is ever subtracted.

ROMAN NUMERALS	ARABIC NUMBERS
IV or iv̈	4
IX or iẍ	9
XL	40

When a numeral of lesser value follows one of greater value, add the one of lesser value to the one of greater value. Only three numerals are ever added.

ROMAN NUMERALS	ARABIC NUMBERS
II or ii	2
VI or vi	6
XV or xv	15
XX or xx	20
XXV or xxv	25
XXX or xxx	30

Roman numerals V, L, and D should never be repeated because it is unnecessary, as shown here:

$$VV = X$$
$$LL = C$$
$$DD = M$$

Sometimes the symbol ss, used to express one half, is used with Roman numerals.

ROMAN NUMBERS	ARABIC NUMBERS
$\overline{ss}$ or $\overset{..}{ss}$ or ss	½
$\overline{iss}$ or $\overset{...}{iss}$ or iss	1½
$\overline{iiss}$ or $\overset{....}{iiss}$ or iiss	2½
$\overline{viiss}$ or $\overset{....}{viiss}$ or viss	7½

MILITARY TIME

More and more hospitals are using military time. Therefore, medication orders are written using military time. The practitioner should be familiar with these time designations. Military time is based on 100 increments of time, beginning with 1:00 AM being designated as 0100 hours and each additional local hour adding an increment of 100 to the initial 0100 base, so that midnight would be 2400 hours. Minute increments are written as in standard time; for example; 1:15 AM would be written as 0115 and 12:30 AM would be written as 2430.

STANDARD TIME	MILITARY TIME
1:00 AM	0100
2:00 AM	0200
3:00 AM	0300
4:00 AM	0400

5:00 AM	0500
6:00 AM	0600
7:00 AM	0700
8:00 AM	0800
9:00 AM	0900
10:00 AM	1000
11:00 AM	1100
12:00 noon	1200
1:00 PM	1300
2:00 PM	1400
3:00 PM	1500
4:00 PM	1600
5:00 PM	1700
6:00 PM	1800
7:00 PM	1900
8:00 PM	2000
9:00 PM	2100
10:00 PM	2200
11:00 PM	2300
12:00 midnight	2400

PART 3 • Arithmetic Practice Problems

Answers can be found in Appendix C, pp. 236–242.

Simplify these complex fractions:

1. $\dfrac{1\frac{1}{2}}{2} =$

2. $\dfrac{1\frac{3}{4}}{2} =$

3. $\dfrac{2\frac{1}{4}}{3} =$

4. $\dfrac{\frac{1}{3}}{1} =$

5. $\dfrac{1\frac{1}{3}}{2} =$

Add these common fractions:

6. $\frac{1}{150} + \frac{1}{300} =$

7. $1\frac{1}{2} + \frac{3}{4} =$

8. $\frac{4}{3} + \frac{3}{2} =$

9. $1\frac{1}{2} + 2\frac{1}{3} =$

10. $\frac{1}{1000} + \frac{1}{1} =$

11. $\frac{2}{1} + \frac{1}{2} =$

12. $\frac{1}{100} + \frac{1}{200} =$

13. $\frac{4}{3} + \frac{5}{4} =$

14. $1\frac{1}{4} + 1\frac{1}{5} =$

15. $3 + \frac{1}{300} =$

Subtract these common fractions:

16. $\frac{1}{150} - \frac{1}{200} =$

17. $\frac{4}{3} - \frac{1}{2} =$

18. $1\frac{1}{2} - 1\frac{1}{4} =$

19. $3 - 1\frac{1}{3} =$

20. $\frac{1}{1000} - \frac{1}{2000} =$

21. $\frac{5}{4} - \frac{1}{3} =$

22. $3\frac{1}{2} - 2\frac{1}{3} =$

23. $100 - 33\frac{1}{3} =$

24. $1000 - 666\frac{2}{3} =$

25. $2 - 1\frac{1}{3} =$

Multiply these common fractions:

26. $\frac{1}{3} \times \frac{1}{2} =$

27. $\frac{3}{2} \times \frac{5}{4} =$

28. $2\frac{1}{3} \times 1\frac{1}{2} =$

29. $2 \times \frac{1}{1000} =$

30. $\frac{1}{8000} \times \frac{1}{1000} =$

31. $\frac{1}{10,000} \times 100 =$

32. $\frac{1}{12,000} \times 1 =$

33. $\frac{1}{8} \times 1\frac{1}{4} =$

34. $\frac{2}{100} \times \frac{3000}{1} =$

35. $1000 \times 1\frac{1}{2} =$

36. $1 \times \frac{1}{120} =$

37. $\frac{1}{4} \times 32 =$

38. $60 \times 1\frac{1}{2} =$

39. $64 \times 1\frac{1}{2} =$

40. $\frac{1}{10,000} \times 1000 =$

41. $\frac{1}{8} \times 30 =$

42. $\frac{1}{8} \times 32 =$

43. $\frac{2}{1} \times \frac{10,000}{1} =$

44. $\frac{1}{8} \times x =$

45. $\frac{1}{1} \times x =$

46. $1 \times \frac{1}{100} =$

47. $\frac{1}{200} \times x =$

48. $64 \times \frac{1}{3} =$

49. $60 \times \frac{1}{3} =$

50. $\frac{5}{100} \times \frac{3000}{1} =$

Divide these common fractions:

51. $\frac{2}{3} \div \frac{3}{4} =$

52. $\frac{1}{4} \div \frac{1}{4} =$

53. $\dfrac{\frac{3}{4}}{\frac{1}{2}} =$

54. $\frac{300}{150} \div \frac{2}{1} =$

55. $\dfrac{\frac{3}{2}}{\frac{2}{1}} =$

56. $1\frac{1}{4} \div 2\frac{1}{3} =$

57. $1000 \div \frac{1}{3} =$

58. $\frac{1000}{12,000} \div \frac{1}{8000} =$

59. $4 \div \frac{40}{1} =$

60. $\frac{1}{8} \div \frac{1}{12,000} =$

61. $\dfrac{1\frac{1}{4}}{2} =$

62. $\frac{1}{200} \div \frac{1}{100} =$

63. $^{1000}/_{10,000} \div {}^{1}/_{1000} =$

64. $\dfrac{1\frac{1}{2}}{2} =$

65. $^{1}/_{200} \div {}^{1}/_{150} =$

66. $^{1000}/_{12,000} \div {}^{1}/_{1} =$

67. $\frac{1}{2} \div 1 =$

68. $100 \div {}^{9}/_{10} =$

69. $30 \div \frac{1}{8} =$

70. $32 \div \frac{1}{8} =$

71. $^{1}/_{120} \div {}^{1}/_{60} =$

72. $64 \div \frac{3}{4} =$

73. $60 \div \frac{3}{4} -$

74. $^{1}/_{150} \div \frac{1}{2} =$

75. $1\frac{2}{3} \div 2 =$

Compare sizes of these fractions:

Which is smaller:

76. $\frac{1}{2}$ or $\frac{1}{3}$?

77. $^{1}/_{150}$ or $^{1}/_{200}$?

78. $^{1}/_{10,000}$ or $^{1}/_{8000}$?

79. $^{1}/_{300}$ or $^{1}/_{150}$?

80. $^{2}/_{300}$ or $^{1}/_{300}$?

81. $^{2}/_{4}$ or $^{4}/_{2}$?

82. $^{1}/_{1}$ or $\frac{1}{2}$?

83. $^{1000}/_{1}$ or $^{500}/_{1}$?

84. $^{1}/_{64}$ or $^{1}/_{60}$?

85. $^{2}/_{1}$ or $^{4}/_{3}$?

Which Is Larger:

86. 3.015 or 3.019?

87. 0.002 or 0.0015?

88. 4.005 or 4.000?

89. 60.40 or 60.35?

90. 100.66 or 100.67?

91. 64.33 or 64.35?

92. 7.5 or 7.45?

93. 1.145 or 1.15?

94. 0.125 or 0.200?

95. 0.0025 or 0.002?

Change these common fractions to decimal fractions:

96. $\frac{1}{2} =$

97. $^{1}/_{200} =$

98. $^{5}/_{100} =$

99. $^{1}/_{100} =$

100. $^{2}/_{100} =$

101. $\frac{3}{4} =$

102. $\frac{2}{3} =$

103. $^{1}/_{10,000} =$

104. $\frac{1}{8} =$

105. $2\frac{1}{4} =$

Change these decimal fractions to common fractions:

106. $0.0001 =$

107. $0.03 =$

108. $0.50 =$

109. $0.01 =$

110. $0.005 =$

111. $0.500 =$

112. $0.27 =$

113. $0.6 =$

114. $1.125 =$

115. $0.25 =$

Round off to the nearest 10th:

116. $4.01 =$

117. $0.056 =$

118. $6.033 =$

119. $5.505 =$

120. $0.075 =$

Round off to the nearest 100th:

121. $2.00875 =$

122. $5.006 =$

123. $0.104 =$

124. $1.0033 =$

125. $0.033 =$

Add these decimals:

126. $0.004 + 0.006 =$

127. $0.5 + 0.25 =$

128. $0.05 + 0.5 =$

129. $0.003 + 0.0006 =$

130. $1.33 + 0.050 =$

Subtract these decimals:

131. $0.06 - 0.004 =$

132. $0.5 - 0.25 =$

133. $0.004 - 0.0005 =$

134. $0.25 - 0.125 =$

135. $0.006 - 0.003 =$

Multiply these decimals:

136. $1.25 \times 0.75 =$

137. $0.5 \times 0.5 =$

138. $0.1 \times 0.01 =$

139. $0.008 \times 1.0 =$

140. $0.001 \times 1.5 =$

Divide these decimals:

141. $1.25 \div 75 =$

142. $0.6 \div 0.03 =$

143. $0.1 \div 0.01 =$

144. $0.5 \div 0.5 =$

145. $0.1 \div 0.005 =$

Change these percents to common fractions:

146. $0.2\% =$

147. $\frac{1}{10}\% =$

148. $15\% =$

149. $100\% =$

150. $0.01\% =$

Change these common fractions to percents:

151. $\frac{1}{8} =$

152. $\frac{1}{10,000} =$

153. $1\frac{1}{2} =$

154. $\frac{1}{100} =$

155. $\frac{1}{500} =$

Change these percents to decimal fractions:

156. $0.1\% =$

157. $2\% =$

158. $50\% =$

159. $0.0125\% =$

160. $100\% =$

Change these decimal fractions to percents:

161. $0.004 =$

162. $3.33 =$

163. $0.9 =$

164. $0.01 =$

165. $6.67 =$

Change these common fractions to ratios:

166. $\frac{1}{60} =$

167. $\frac{1000}{1} =$

168. $1\frac{2}{3} =$

169. $\frac{5}{10,000} =$

170. $1\frac{3}{4} =$

Change these ratios to common fractions:

171. $1:1000 =$

172. $5:100 =$

173. $0.4:1000 =$

174. $1:1.5 =$

175. $1:0.05 =$

Change these decimal fractions to ratios:

176. $0.25 =$

177. $0.001 =$

178. $5.5 =$

179. $0.8 =$

180. $0.05 =$

Change these ratios to decimal fractions:

181. $1:10,000 =$

182. $5:1000 =$

183. $1:0.9 =$

184. $1:0.01 =$

185. $100:0.001 =$

Change these percents to ratios:

186. $0.9\% =$

187. $0.5\% =$

188. 10% =

189. 3% =

190. 100% =

Change these ratios to percents:

191. $1:0.05 =$

192. $100:5000 =$

193. $1:60 =$

194. $5:100 =$

195. $1:0.001 =$

Determine the unknown mean in ratio and proportion:

196. $5:100 = x:60$

197. $2:100 = x:1000$

198. $10:x = 0.5:10{,}000$

199. $16:x = 40:16$

200. $^2/_{100}:^1/_2 = x:3000$

201. $1000:x = 125:1$

202. $0.5:x = 0.3:1$

203. $300{,}000:x = 150{,}000:5$

204. $0.5:x = 0.25:1$

205. $^1/_{12{,}000}:^1/_{8000} = x:1000$

Determine the unknown extreme in ratio and proportion

206. $16:1000 = 1:x$

207. $1:60 = 1\frac{1}{2}:x$

208. $60:1 = 15:x$

209. $x:100 = 30:600$

210. $^1/_{10{,}000}:^1/_1 = 30:x$

211. $80:16 = 18:x$

212. $125:1 = 1000:x$

213. $300{,}000:1 = 3{,}000{,}000:x$

214. $0.3:1 = 0.5:x$

215. $^1/_{150}:1 = ^1/_{200}:x$

Convert °F to °C:

216. 212°F =

217. 32°F =

218. 82°F =

219. 0°F =

220. 60°F =

Convert °C to °F:

221. 0°C =

222. 100°C =

223. 20°C =

224. 35°C =

225. 40°C =

Change these Roman numerals to Arabic numbers:

226. IXX =

227. vii =

228. XC =

229. xvi =

230. LX =

Change these Arabic numbers to Roman numerals:

231. 4 =

232. 12 =

233. 8 =

234. 1000 =

235. 150 =

Change standard time to military time:

236. 12:00 noon =

237. 1:45 AM =

238. 3:15 PM =

239. 12:30 AM =

240. 2:10 PM =

Change military time to standard time:

241. 2400 =

242. 0320 =

243. 1810 =

244. 1650 =

245. 1100 =

PART 4 • Arithmetic Review Problems

Answers can be found in Appendix C, pp. 242–245.

Which is larger:

1. $\frac{1}{300}$ or $\frac{1}{150}$?

2. 0.5% or $\frac{1}{5}$%?

3. $\frac{1}{12,000}$ or $\frac{1}{8000}$?

4. 0.006 or 0.03?

5. 0.5 or 0.25?

Which is smaller:

6. $\frac{3}{1000}$ or $\frac{2}{1000}$?

7. 1.27 or 1.266?

8. 10.745 or 10.75?

9. 5.025 or 5.0245?

10. 2.66 or 2.667?

Change to common fractions:

11. 0.0125 =

12. 0.4% =

13. 1:10,000 =

Change to decimal fractions:

14. 8%

15. 1:100

16. $\frac{1}{25}$

Change to ratios:

17. 2.5

18. $\frac{1}{10,000}$

19. 0.2%

Change to percent:

20. 0.125

21. $\frac{1}{150}$

22. 1:10,000

Round off to the nearest 1000th:

23. $0.333\frac{1}{3}$

24. $0.6\frac{2}{3}$

25. $1\frac{1}{3}$

Complete the following:

26. $\frac{1}{300} + \frac{1}{150} =$

27. $\frac{2}{3} + \frac{3}{2} =$

28. $0.025 \div 1000 =$

29. $0.002 \div 0.004 =$

30. $\dfrac{1\frac{2}{3}}{2} =$

31. $\frac{1}{4} \div \frac{1}{8000} =$

32. $\frac{4}{2} \times \frac{3}{4} =$

33. $0.5 \div 0.3 =$

34. $10 \div 0.05 =$

35. $\frac{3}{2} \div \frac{1}{2} =$

36. $2 - 0.05 =$

37. $1\frac{3}{4} \times 0.05 =$

38. $\dfrac{\frac{2}{3}}{1} =$

39. $60 \times \frac{1}{3} =$

40. $500 - \frac{1}{3} =$

41. $1.5 \div 0.25 =$

42. $1000 - 666\frac{2}{3} =$

43. $1000 \times 0.05 =$

44. $0.5 \times \frac{1}{200} =$

45. $1\frac{1}{3} + \frac{1}{4} =$

46. $0.005 \div 1000 =$

47. $\frac{1}{150} - \frac{1}{300} =$

48. $\frac{1}{10,000} \times 500 =$

49. $2\frac{2}{3} + 1\frac{3}{4} =$

50. $\frac{5}{2} - \frac{2}{3} =$

51. $5\frac{1}{5} - 2\frac{1}{4} =$

52. $2\frac{2}{3} \times 1\frac{1}{2} =$

53. $7\frac{1}{2} \times \frac{1}{4} =$

54. $60 \div \frac{1}{4} =$

Round off to the nearest 10th:

55. $0.133 =$

56. $1.266 =$

57. $4.505 =$

Round off to the nearest 100th:

58. $0.666 =$

59. $1.003 =$

60. $5.0125 =$

Solve for x, the unknown value:

61. $15:1 = x:0.5$

62. $1000:1 = 0.025:x$

63. $80:16 = 30:x$

64. $1:60 = x:32$

65. $\frac{1}{3}:1 = x:30$

66. $0.5:1 = 10:x$

67. $\frac{1}{12,000}:\frac{1}{8000} = x:3000$

68. $200,000:1 = 1,000,000:x$

69. $1:1000 = 0.5:x$

70. $0.004:1 = 0.002:x$

Change to Arabic numbers:

71. $\dot{\overline{\text{iv}}} =$

72. $\overset{\cdots}{\text{iss}} =$

73. $\text{XII} -$

74. $\text{ii} =$

75. $\text{M} =$

76. $\text{XXX} =$

77. $\text{xv} =$

78. $\overset{\cdots}{\overline{\text{viiss}}} =$

79. $\text{CXX} =$

80. $\text{XV} =$

Change to Roman numerals:

81. $1\frac{1}{2} =$

82. $30 =$

83. $1000 =$

84. $7\frac{1}{2} =$

85. $15 =$

86. $90 =$

87. $4 =$

88. $60 =$

89. $400 =$

90. $2500 =$

Convert °F to °C:

91. $98.6°F =$

92. $200°F =$

93. $-50°F =$

94. $10°F =$

95. $68°F =$

Convert °C to °F:

96. $38°C =$

97. $43°C =$

98. $10°C =$

99. $34°C =$

100. $-10°C =$

Change standard time to military time:

101. 12:30 AM =

102. 4:20 PM =

103. 10:15 AM =

104. 7:30 AM =

105. 9:00 PM =

Change military time to standard time:

106. 2400 =

107. $0800 =$ 109. $1530 =$

108. $2100 =$ 110. $0910 =$

PART 5 • Arithmetic Post-Test

Answers can be found in Appendix C, pp. 245–247.

1. Which is larger, $\frac{1}{150}$ or $\frac{1}{300}$?

2. $\frac{2}{3} + \frac{1}{4} =$

3. Change $\frac{1}{100}$ to a decimal fraction.

4. Change 0.125% to a ratio.

5. Change $1:1000$ to a percent.

6. Round off 0.66 to the nearest 10th.

7. Solve for x when $60:1 = x:0.50$.

8. Convert 98°F to °C.

9. Change IX to an Arabic number.

10. $1\frac{1}{2} \div \frac{1}{2} =$

11. $\frac{1}{60} \times 4 =$

12. Which is smaller, 0.006 or 0.03?

13. Change 3% to a ratio.

14. Solve for x when $2x = \frac{300}{150}$.

15. Convert 9°C to °F.

16. Change $7\frac{1}{2}$ to a Roman numeral.

17. $0.33 - 0.033 =$

18. Solve for x when $200,000:2 = 300,000:x$.

19. $8\frac{1}{3} \times 15 =$

20. Change $7\frac{1}{2}$ to a percent.

21. Solve for x when $125:5 = 0.25:x$.

22. Solve for x when $1:1000 = 0.005:x$.

23. Change 5% to a decimal fraction.

24. Solve for x when $0.25:5 = 0.3:x$.

25. $1500 \div 4 =$

26. Solve for x when $\frac{1}{64}:1 = x:32$.

27. Change 0.667 to a percent.

28. $\dfrac{0.3 \times 500}{1.7} =$

29. $\dfrac{8}{8+12} \times 500 =$

30. Solve for x when $1:64 = 1\frac{1}{2}:x$.

31. Which is larger, $\frac{1}{10}\%$ or $\frac{1}{20}\%$?

32. Change 50% to a ratio.

33. Solve for x when $1:15 = 8\frac{1}{3}:x$.

34. Change 0.5% to a ratio.

35. $3000 \div 24 =$

36. Round off $0.666\frac{2}{3}$ to the nearest 100th.

37. Solve for x when $\frac{1}{60}:1 = x:2$.

38. Which is larger, $\frac{1}{200}$, $\frac{1}{150}$, or $\frac{1}{120}$?

39. Change 2:1000 to a decimal fraction.

40. Solve for x when 4:1 = x:2.

41. Which is smaller, 1:1000 or 1:100?

42. Solve for x when 0.25:1 = 0.5:x.

43. Solve for x when 15:1 = x:0.3.

44. Which is larger, 1:1000 or 1:100?

45. Change $\frac{1}{150}$ to a percent.

46. Solve for x when 0.01:1 = x:5.

47. Solve for x when 2.2:1 = 18:x.

48. $\dfrac{0.44 \times 0.5}{1.7} =$

49. Solve for x when 80:1 = x:1.3.

50. Solve for x when 100:16 = 40:x.

51. Change 2400 to standard time.

52. Change 10:00 PM to military time.

53. Change 2010 to standard time.

54. Change 4:00 PM to military time.

55. Change 1300 to standard time.

56. Which is larger, $\frac{1}{150}$ or $\frac{1}{300}$?

57. $\frac{1}{100} + \frac{2}{1000} =$

58. $1\frac{1}{2} - \frac{4}{3} =$

59. $2\frac{1}{2} - 1\frac{1}{5} =$

60. $6\frac{1}{3} - \frac{1}{6} =$

61. $\frac{60}{4} \times \frac{15}{1} =$

62. $\frac{64}{2} \div \frac{16}{2} =$

63. Change 0.025 to a common fraction.

64. Which is larger, 0.66 or 0.7?

65. Which is smaller, 0.66 or 0.667?

66. Change 0.2% to a common fraction.

67. Change 0.01% to a ratio.

68. Change 1.125 to a ratio.

69. $0.01 \times 1000 =$

70. $2.875 : 0.05 =$

CHAPTER 2

Overview

OBJECTIVES

At the end of this chapter, the student should be able to:
- Recall the more common equivalents from the apothecaries', metric, and household systems of measurement
- Recall the common abbreviations used in medication orders
- Use Formula A to convert dosages from one system of measurement to another system of measurement
- Understand the use of Formula B in the calculation of most medication dosages

---

PART 6 • Introduction

In most hospitals, the pharmacy provides medications in what is called a "unit dose." This means that drugs are available to the practitioner in the exact amount ordered to be given. Therefore, little or no calculation of dosages is necessary.

However, on specialty units in most hospitals, such as the emergency room, intensive care unit, and coronary care unit, practitioners must calculate and prepare many medications. In most small hospitals, they must do so on all units.

Working dosage problems involves the calculation of the correct dosage to be administered to the patient, usually either orally or parenterally, in order to give the prescribed amount of a drug. Usually the physician orders the drug in numbers of grains, grams, or other units of *weight* measure. To administer the correct dosage, one often needs to convert this order to a number of tablets, capsules, minims, drams, ounces, milliliters, or other units of *volume* or *capacity* measure. A single ratio and proportion formula (hereafter referred to as Formula B) can be used to work most dosage problems.

Doing solutions problems involves determining how to prepare solutions, for either oral or topical use. There are two variations of solution problems, but both can be solved by using Formula B.

In solving either dosage or solution problems, a second ratio and proportion formula (hereafter referred to as Formula A) may be used to determine equivalent values whenever necessary. This additional initial step may be necessary in order to limit the different units of measure in any proportion to two units of measure. One can say, for example, that 4 wheels:1 car = 8 wheels:2 cars. One cannot say, however, that 4 wheels:1 car = 8 wheels:2 bicycles. Therefore, if the physician orders aspirin grains x (10) and the available tablets are labeled "0.3 gram," Formula A would be used first to convert either grains x to its gram equivalent or to convert 0.3 grams to its grain equivalent. Then, when using Formula B to determine how many tablets to give, tablets would be one unit of measure and either grains or grams would be the other unit of measure. A grain is an apothecaries' system of measure; a gram is a metric system of measure.

PART 7 • Systems of Measurement

The American colonists brought to this country the use of the apothecaries' system of weight and measures, which was then being used in England. England has adopted the use of the metric system, which has long been the single lawful system in most European countries. Since World War II, there has been a growing tendency in the United States for doctors to order drugs and pharmaceutical companies to label drugs with the metric system units of measure. Learning to administer drugs would be greatly simplified if only the metric system were used. Until that time, however, one needs to know about three systems of measurement: the apothecaries', the metric, and the household systems. Tables and explanations of these three systems and approximate equivalents among the systems may be found farther on. More detailed and/or exact apothecaries' and metric system equivalents can be found in Appendix A.

One thing should be emphasized before anyone becomes discouraged from consulting these lengthy tables. Almost all the equivalents that health-care professionals will ever need to know can be determined by using ratio and proportion with the few equivalents listed in Table 2–5, page 36.

APOTHECARIES' SYSTEM

The apothecaries' system is one of several different and confusing old English systems of weights and measurements. The basic unit of weight in the apothecaries' system is the *grain,* originally the weight of 1 grain of wheat. The basic unit of fluid measure in this system is the *minim,* the approximate amount of water that would weigh 1 grain. Other units of measure from this system that may be used in drug administration are given in Table 2–1. Additional apothecaries' units of measure that are rarely or never used by practitioners in the administration of drugs can be found in Appendix A.

Sometimes symbols are used to express apothecaries' units of measure. The most commonly used apothecaries' symbols are ℨ for dram and ℥ for ounce. Also, when using the apothecaries' units, the numerical value or the quantity of a unit is often expressed in Roman numerals, usually in lowercase letters. For example, 5 grains may be written as "grains v," 4 drams as "ℨiv," and 6 ounces as "℥vi." It is customary to use regular fractions such as ½ or ¼ for the apothecaries' system rather than decimal fractions such as 0.5 or 0.25.

TABLE 2–1 • **Apothecaries'** Equivalents	
Weight Units	
60 grains (gr)	1 dram (ℨ or dr)
8 drams (ℨ) or 480 grains	1 ounce (ℨ)
12 ounces (ℨ)	1 pound (lb)
Fluid Units	
60 minims (m)	1 fluid dram (flℨ)
8 fluid drams (flℨ) or 480 minims (m)	1 fluid ounce (flℨ)
16 fluid ounces (flℨ)	1 pint (pt or O)
2 pints (pt or O)	1 quart (qt)
4 quarts (qt)	1 gallon (C or gal)
*Weight Units**	*Fluid Units**
1 grain (gr)	1 minim (m)
60 grains (gr)	1 fluid dram (flℨ), 60 m
480 grains (gr)	1 fluid ounce (flℨ), 480 m

*The above apothecaries' weight-fluid units are approximate equivalents only but, when needed, these approximations are acceptable for the preparation and administration of solutions and drugs.

METRIC SYSTEM

During the latter part of the 18th century, the French devised the metric system based upon the decimal system and unalterable standards of measurement. Then, in 1875, the International Bureau of Weights and Measures was established in Paris by the International Metric Convention. This bureau prepared international standards for the participating countries.

The metric units of measurements are the *gram* (weight), the *liter* (volume), and the *meter* (linear). These basic units can be divided by or multiplied by 10, 100, or 1000. Latin prefixes are used to designate the subdivisions of these units and Greek prefixes are used to designate multiples of these units, as shown here for the gram (g):

$$
\begin{aligned}
1 \text{ kilogram (kg)} &= 1000.0 \ \text{g} \\
1 \text{ hectogram (hg)} &= 100.0 \ \text{g} \\
1 \text{ dekagram (dkg)} &= 10.0 \ \text{g} \\
1 \text{ gram (g)} &= 1.0 \ \text{g} \\
1 \text{ decigram (dg)} &= 0.1 \ \text{g} \\
1 \text{ centigram (cg)} &= 0.01 \ \text{g} \\
1 \text{ milligram (mg)} &= 0.001 \ \text{g}
\end{aligned}
$$

The metric system of measurement is used throughout most of the world. Its use, especially in drug administration, is becoming prevalent in the United States. Decimal fractions are used for the metric system. To minimize the danger of an error, a zero is placed before the decimal point when writing a fraction of a metric unit.

Gram

The gram, the basic metric unit of weight used in pharmaceutical weighing of drugs, is equal to the weight of 1 milliliter (mL) of distilled water at 4° on the Celsius (C) scale. The kilogram (1 kg or 1000 g) is the only multiple of the gram used by health-care workers. It may be used to calculate drug dosages, fluid requirements, and so forth, in terms of kilograms of body weight. The only subdivisions of a gram commonly used are the milligram (mg or 0.001 g) and the microgram (mcg or 0.001 mg).

$$1 \text{ kilogram (kg)} = 1000 \text{ grams (g)}$$
$$1 \text{ gram (g)} = 1000 \text{ milligrams (mg)}$$
$$1 \text{ milligram (mg)} = 1000 \text{ micrograms (mcg)}$$

The abbreviation ''μg'' may be used on drug labels for micrograms but when written it could be confused with ''mg'' for milligrams, a quantity 1000 times greater. It is safer to use the abbreviation ''mcg.''

Liter

The liter, the metric volume unit that is very frequently used by health-care practitioners, is equal to the contents of 1 decimeter (10 centimeters) cube. The liter was found to be 1000.028 cubic centimeters (cc) rather than the 1000 cc intended. A liter does contain 1000 milliliters (mL). Even though a cubic centimeter is 0.000028 cc less than a milliliter, in drug administration a cubic centimeter and a milliliter are considered to be equal and are used interchangeably.

Since a gram is equal to the weight of 1 milliliter of distilled water at 4°C, 1 gram equals 1 milliliter is an equivalent that may be used in the calculations needed to prepare some oral and topical solutions. This equivalent is an approximate one, not an accurate one, when used for such purposes.

$$1 \text{ liter (L)} = 1000 \text{ milliliters (mL)}$$

Meter

The meter, the metric linear unit of measurement, is 39.37 inches. Centimeters, millimeters, and, occasionally, microns (one thousandth of a millimeter) are the only linear metric measures used by health care personnel. There are approximately 2.5 centimeters per 1 inch. The sides of a cubic centimeter are approximately 0.4 of an inch each.

$$1 \text{ meter (m)} = 1000 \text{ millimeters (mm)}$$

Table 2–2 gives the commonly used metric equivalents.

HOUSEHOLD MEASURES

Practitioners may use or teach the use of household articles for the measurements of drugs or solutions of drugs. Because household measurements are not accurate, ordinarily one should not substitute household equivalents or metric or apothecaries' measurements ordered by the physician. Note that all household measures are volume measurements. Occasionally, however, a volume measure must be used as a substitute for a weight measure. The equivalents in Table 2–3 are approximate, not accurate. Occasionally household measures are used for ordering dosages of medications. The quantity may be written in either Arabic or Roman numerals. For example, 15 drops

TABLE 2–2 • **Metric Equivalents**	
Weight Units	
1 kilogram (kg)	1000 grams (g)
1 gram (g)	1000 milligrams (mg)
1 milligram (mg)	1000 micrograms (mcg)
Fluid Units	
1 liter (L)	1000 milliliters (mL)
*Weight Units**	*Fluid Units**
1 gram (g)	1 milliliter (mL)
1000 grams (g)	1 liter (L)
Linear Units	
1 meter (m)	10 decimeters (dm)
1 decimeter (dm)	10 centimeters (cm)
1 centimeter (cm)	10 millimeters (mm)

*The above metric weight-fluid units are approximate equivalents only but, when needed, these approximations are acceptable for the preparation and administration of solutions and drugs.

TABLE 2–3 • **Approximate Household Equivalents**	
Household	*Household*
15–16 drops (gtts)	¼ teaspoon (tsp)
2 teaspoons	1 dessertspoon (dssp)
3 teaspoons	1 tablespoon (Tbsp)
2 tablespoons	1 fluid ounce (fl oz)
3 dessertspoons	1 fluid ounce
6 fluid ounces	1 teacup
8 fluid ounces	1 glass or 1 measuring cup

may be written as "15 gtts" or as "gtts xv." "Gtts" is an acceptable abbreviation for drops.

MEASUREMENT EQUIVALENTS

Table 2–4 contains approximate household, apothecaries', and metric equivalents that are of particular value when helping patients transfer the more specific apothecaries' or metric physician's order into measurements that they can find in their households. The most frequently used weight and volume equivalents are shown in Table 2–5. Memorization of the few equivalents in this table enables one to determine most other system equivalents.

TABLE 2–4 • Approximate Household, Apothecaries', and Metric Equivalents

Household	Apothecaries'	Metric
1 drop	1 minim	0.06–0.07 mL
1 teaspoon	1 fluid dram	4 or 5 mL
1 tablespoon	4 fluid drams	15 or 16 mL
2 tablespoons	1 fluid ounce	30 or 32 mL
3 dessertspoons	1 fluid ounce	30 or 32 mL
1 teacup	6 fluid ounces	180 or 192 mL
1 glass or 1 measuring cup	8 fluid ounces or ½ pint	240 or 250 mL
2 glasses or 2 measuring cups	16 fluid ounces or 1 pint	480 or 500 mL
4 glasses or 4 measuring cups	1 quart	960 or 1000 mL

TABLE 2–5 • Most Frequently Used Approximate Equivalents

Weight Units			Fluid Units		
House-hold =	Metric =	Apothecaries'	House-hold =	Metric =	Apothecaries'
1 g or 1,000 mg or 1,000,000 mcg		15–16 gr	15 or 16 gtts	1 mL	15 or 16 m
	60, 64, or 65 mg	1 gr			
2 Tbsp or 3 dssp or 6 tsp	30 or 32 g	1 oz or 8 dr	2 Tbsp or 3 dssp or 6 tsp	30 or 32 mL	1 fl oz or 8 fl dr
			2 glasses	500 mL	1 pt or 16 fl oz
1 kg or 1000 g	2.2 or 2.3 lb (imperial or avoir-dupois, not apothecaries')		4 glasses	1000 mL or 1 L	1 qt
				4000 mL	1 gal

Additional approximate and exact apothecaries' and metric volume and weight equivalents may be found in tables in Appendix A.

PART 8 • Other Abbreviations

SYSTÈME INTERNATIONAL (SI) AND OTHER ABBREVIATIONS

Metric measure abbreviations presented thus far are the official International System of Units (IU), or the French Système International d'Unités (SI), abbreviations that are now in use.

Older abbreviations of metric units of measurement that one can expect to see in physician's orders and on drug labels for some time to come are as follows:

$$gram = Gm$$
$$milliliter = ml$$
$$meter = M$$
$$cubic\ centimeter = cc$$

DRUG ADMINISTRATION

Table 2–6 contains common abbreviations used by physicians in ordering medications and by practitioners in administering drugs. These abbreviations should be memorized. In addition to this list of abbreviations, each individual hospital or geographic region may have additional and/or different abbreviations acceptable to the specific hospital or region. Those abbreviations, as well as the ones presented here, should be memorized.

TABLE 2–6 • Abbreviations Used in Drug Administration			
Abbreviation	**Meaning**	**Abbreviation**	**Meaning**
a̅a̅	of each	os	mouth
ac	before meals	OU	both eyes
ad lib	as desired	oz	ounce
aq	water	pc	after meals
aq dist or DW	distilled water	per	by
bid	twice a day	PO or per os	by mouth
c̅	with	prn	when required
caps	capsules	qh	every hour
comp	compound	q2h	every 2 hours
dil	dilute	q3h	every 3 hours
elix	elixir	q4h	every 4 hours
ext	extract	qid	four times a day
fld or fl	fluid	qod	every other day
g or Gm	gram	qoh	every other hour
gr	grain	qs	quantity sufficient
gtt	drop	℞	take
H	by hypodermic	s̅	without
h or hr	hour	SC or sc	subcutaneously
hs	hour of sleep	Sig or S	write on label
IM	intramuscularly	sol	solution
IV	intravenously	sos	once if necessary
kg	kilogram	sp	spirits
m	minim	s̅s̅	a half
n, noc, or noct	night	stat	immediately
non rep	not to be repeated	supp	suppository
NPO	nothing by mouth	syr	syrup
ol	oil	tid	three times a day
OD	right eye	tr or tinct	tincture
od or qd	every day	U	unit
om or qam	every morning	ung	ointment
on or qpm	every night	vin	wine
OS	left eye		

PART 9 • Methods of Calculation

RATIO AND PROPORTION

A ratio is the same as a fraction and can be expressed in algebraic form (1:2) or as a regular fraction (½). Either way, the relationship is stated as "one is to two."

A proportion is an equation of equal fractions or ratios. For example, the ratios ½ and ⁴⁄₈ are equal, or "one is to two as four is to eight" (1:2::4:8) or "one is to two equals four is to eight" (1:2=4:8).

The first and fourth terms of a proportion are called the *extremes* and the second and third terms are called the *means*. In solving these equations, the product of the means equals the product of the extremes.

$$\text{First term : Second term} = \text{Third term : Fourth term}$$

Means (Second term, Third term)

Extremes (First term, Fourth term)

or

$$2 \times 4 = 8$$
Means

$$1:2 = 4:8$$
Extremes

$$1 \times 8 = 8$$

The terms of the two ratios of a proportion must correspond in relative value. For example, small is to small as large is to large, or small is to large as small is to large.

$$1:2 = 4:8 \quad \text{small : small} = \text{large : large?}$$
$$\text{or}$$
$$1:4 = 2:8 \quad \text{small : large} = \text{small : large?}$$

This correspondence, which is confusing enough when only numerical values are used, is more confusing when numerical values plus two units of measure are involved, as in dosage and solutions problems. For example, if 15 grains (gr) equals 1 gram (g), 30 gr equals how many grams?

$$15 \text{ gr}:1 \text{ g} = 30 \text{ gr}:x \text{ g}$$
$$15 \text{ x} = 30$$
$$x = 2 \text{ g; therefore, 30 gr equals 2 g}$$
$$\text{or}$$
$$15 \text{ gr}:1 \text{ g} = 30 \text{ gr}:2 \text{ g}$$

Disregarding numerical values, the ratios in this proportion correspond— small : large = small : large—because grains are smaller units of measure than grams. However, the numerical values cannot be disregarded. Both the relative value of the units of measure and the relative value of the quantities of these units of measurement must be considered. Otherwise, even when using the correct measurement values, the product of the means *may not equal* the product of the extremes, as shown here:

$$\text{Product of means} = \quad 2 \times 30 = 60$$
$$15 \text{ gr} : 2 \text{ g} = 30 \text{ gr} : 1 \text{ g}$$
$$\text{Product of extremes} = \quad 15 \times 1 = 15$$

Unless the proportion is stated properly, the solution to the problem will be *incorrect,* as shown in the previous and following example:

$$15 \text{ gr} : x \text{ g} = 30 \text{ gr} : 1 \text{ g}$$
$$30 \text{ x} = 15$$
$$x = 0.5 \text{ g}$$

Therefore, 15 gr equals 0.5 g, which is *incorrect.*

There are many possible ways to state *correctly* this one proportion, using the underlined known value of 15 gr = 1 g:

$$\underline{15 \text{ gr} : 1 \text{ g}} = 30 \text{ gr} : x \text{ g}$$
or
$$\underline{15 \text{ gr}} : 30 \text{ gr} = \underline{1 \text{ g}} : x \text{ g}$$
or
$$\underline{1 \text{ g} : 15 \text{ gr}} = x \text{ g} : 30 \text{ gr}$$
or
$$1 \text{ g} : x \text{ g} = \underline{15 \text{ gr}} : 30 \text{ gr}$$
or
$$30 \text{ gr} : x \text{ g} = \underline{15 \text{ gr} : 1 \text{ g}}$$
or
$$30 \text{ gr} : \underline{15 \text{ gr}} = x \text{ g} : \underline{1 \text{ g}}$$
or
$$x \text{ g} : 30 \text{ gr} = \underline{1 \text{ g} : 15 \text{ gr}}$$
or
$$x \text{ g} : \underline{1 \text{ g}} = 30 \text{ gr} : \underline{15 \text{ gr}}$$

There are just as many ways to state *incorrectly* any one proportion.

KNOWN VALUE FORMULAS

To avoid confusion, start every proportion with a ratio of two known values; for example, 15 grains : 1 gram (known equivalents) or 5 grains : 1 tablet (dosage in a certain unit of measure that is *known* to be available for administration).

Next, when using Formulas A and B, make certain that the unit of measure of the third term is the same as that in the first term and that the unit of measure of the fourth term is the same as that in the second term:

FORMULA A   **KNOWN EQUIVALENTS**

(**CONVERSIONS**)   15 gr : 1 g = x gr : 0.5 g

FORMULA B   **KNOWN AMOUNTS**

(**DOSAGES**)   5 gr : 1 tablet = 15 gr : x tablet(s)

As stated above, in all dosages and solutions problems there may be two, but no more than two, different units of measure in addition to numerical values. Label every term in the proportion with a unit of measure. Disregard these units of measure when multiplying means and extremes. Finally, label x, the unknown quantity, with the appropriate unit of measure.

Example Problems

Problem 1: Determine the grain equivalent of 0.5 g.

Solution: FORMULA A

KNOWN EQUIVALENTS   UNKNOWN EQUIVALENTS

$$15 \text{ gr} : 1 \text{ g} = x \text{ gr} : 0.5 \text{ g}$$
$$1 \ x = 7\frac{1}{2}$$
$$x = 7\frac{1}{2} \text{ gr}$$

Problem 2: Determine how many tablets to administer when the order is for aspirin gr xv and the available tablets are gr v each.

Solution: FORMULA B

KNOWN AMOUNTS   UNKNOWN AMOUNTS
(AVAILABLE FOR USE)   (ORDERED)   (NEEDED)

$$\text{dosage} : \text{amount} = \text{dosage} : \text{amount}$$
$$5 \text{ gr} : 1 \text{ tablet} = 15 \text{ gr} : x \text{ tablet(s)}$$
$$5 \ x = 15$$
$$x = 3 \text{ tablets}$$

Note that the first ratio or the first and the second terms in the proportion above are all *known* values. By using the few equivalents listed in Table 2–5 and Formula A, one can determine almost all other equivalents one will ever need to use. Most dosage and solutions problems can be solved by using variations of Formula B.

ALTERNATE WAYS OF CALCULATION

Other methods of setting up the ratios may be used by those who are more familiar with one of these alternate methods. One of the most commonly used alternative methods is to state the first and third terms of the previous method as numerators and the second and fourth terms as denominators. In other words, the ratios are expressed as regular fractions. For example, 15 gr:1000 milligrams (mg) = x gr:100 mg can be shown as follows:

KNOWN EQUIVALENTS $\left[\dfrac{15 \text{ gr}}{1000 \text{ mg}} = \dfrac{x \text{ gr}}{100 \text{ mg}} \right]$ **UNKNOWN EQUIVALENTS**

$$1000 \ x = 1500$$
$$x = 1.5 \text{ or } 1\frac{1}{2} \text{ gr}$$

Or, 5 grains is to 1 tablet as 15 grains is to how many tablets?

KNOWN AMOUNTS $\left[\dfrac{5 \text{ gr}}{1 \text{ tablet}} = \dfrac{15 \text{ gr}}{x \text{ tablets}} \right]$ **UNKNOWN AMOUNTS**

$$5 \ x = 15$$
$$x = 3 \text{ tablets}$$

To solve these fractional equations, cross multiply diagonally. Whichever way the ratios are stated, the product of the means equals the product of the extremes.

Means

$$15 \text{ gr} : 1000 \text{ mg} = x \text{ gr} : 100 \text{ mg}$$

Extremes

or

Extreme   15 gr ↖   ↗ x gr   Mean
=
Mean   1000 mg ↙   ↘ 100 mg   Extreme

Some may prefer to use one of the several variations of the formula of *desired dose over the available dose times the unit of measurement of the available dose equals the amount to give*. The unit of measurement of the available dose is the numerator, usually over an implied denominator of 1. This method will not be used in this book because we have found that users make more errors with this method, especially, for example, when the available dose is available in more than or less than 1 milliliter (mL). It is included as a review for those who have already learned this way of solving problems.

1. $\dfrac{\text{Ordered dose}}{\text{Available dose}} \times \dfrac{\text{Unit of measure}}{\text{of available dose}} = \begin{array}{l}\text{Amount to give} \\ \text{in same unit of} \\ \text{measurement}\end{array}$

ORDERED: 15 gr
AVAILABLE: 5 gr tablets

$$\frac{15 \text{ gr}}{5 \text{ gr}} \times 1 \text{ tablet} = \text{Amount to give}$$

$$\frac{15 \text{ gr}}{5 \text{ gr}} \times \frac{1 \text{ tablet}}{1} = \text{Amount to give}$$

$$\frac{15}{5} = 3 \text{ tablets}$$

2. $\dfrac{\text{D (desired dose)}}{\text{H (on-hand dose)}} \times \text{Quantity} = \text{Amount to give}$

ORDERED: 15 gr
AVAILABLE: 5 gr tablet

$$\frac{15 \text{ gr}}{5 \text{ gr}} \times \frac{1 \text{ tablet}}{1} = ? \text{ tablets}$$

$$\frac{15}{5} = 3 \text{ tablets}$$

3. $\dfrac{\text{Dose ordered}}{\text{Dose on hand}} \times \text{Drug form} = \text{Amount to give}$

ORDERED: 10 mg
AVAILABLE: 40 mg in 2 mL

$$\frac{10 \text{ mg}}{40 \text{ mg}} \times 2 \text{ mL} = \text{Amount to give}$$

$$\frac{20}{40} = 0.5 \text{ mL}$$

DETERMINING EQUIVALENT VALUES WITH FORMULA A

Eight examples of determining equivalent values by using Formula A are presented in the next section, along with discussions of commonly encountered problems. Additional help in determining equivalents is presented later with the answers to the various types of dosage and solutions problems. Formula B will not be used to solve problems until Chapter 3.

Example Problems

Problem 1: 1 gr = ? mg

Solution 1:

KNOWN EQUIVALENTS   UNKNOWN EQUIVALENTS

$$15 \text{ gr}:1000 \text{ mg} = 1 \text{ gr}:x \text{ mg}$$
$$15 \text{ x} = 1000$$
$$x = 66.67 \text{ mg}$$

Solution 2:

$$16 \text{ gr}:1000 \text{ mg} = 1 \text{ gr}:x \text{ mg}$$
$$16x = 1000$$
$$1 = 62.5 \text{ mg}$$

If one remembers the equivalent of 1 gr = 60, 64, or 65 mg from the equivalents given in Table 2–5 and also that 15 or 16 gr = 1 g = 1000 mg, one can see that 1 gr = 60, 64, or 65 mg and that 1 mg = $\frac{1}{60}$, $\frac{1}{64}$, or $\frac{1}{65}$ gr.

$$
\begin{array}{rcl}
1 \text{ g} = & 1000 \text{ mg} = & 15 \text{ or } 16 \text{ gr} \\
& 60, 64, \text{ or } 65 \text{ mg} = & 1 \text{ gr} \\
& 1 \text{ mg} = & \frac{1}{60}, \frac{1}{64}, \text{ or } \frac{1}{65} \text{ gr}
\end{array}
$$

There are a few basic rules that apply to all problems. One is that *no more than a 10 percent margin of difference between the dosage that has been ordered and what is available to be administered can be considered as a safe dosage.* Therefore, any of these values is accurate enough (within the acceptable 10 percent margin of error) for the calculation of dosages. Often the choice of one equivalent over the other two enables division of the numerators and denominators by the same number in order to reduce these to smaller numerical values which are more likely to be the same values as the ordered dosage.

Problem 2: 32 mg = ? gr

Solution 1:

$$1 \text{ gr}:64 \text{ mg} = x \text{ gr}:32 \text{ mg}$$
$$64 \text{ x} = 32$$
$$x = \frac{32}{64}$$
$$x = \frac{1}{2} \text{ gr}$$

Solution 2:

$$1 \text{ gr}:60 \text{ mg} = x \text{ gr}:32 \text{ mg}$$
$$60 \text{ x} = 32$$
$$x = \frac{32}{60}$$
$$x = \frac{8}{15} \text{ gr}$$

If the physician's order is for 32 mg of a certain drug and the tablets are labeled in gr, use 1 gr:64 mg = x gr:32 mg, thus allowing easy reduction of the resulting fraction.

If the physician's order is for 30 mg of this drug, use 1 gr:60 mg = x gr:30 mg, because whether the physician orders 30 mg or 32 mg, the available tablets may be labeled "gr ½." Of course, the tablets may be labeled "30 mg," or "32 mg,' or possibly "0.03 g" or "0.032 g."

Problem 3: Nembutal 100 mg = Nembutal ? gr

Solution 1:
$$15 \text{ gr}:1000 \text{ mg} = x \text{ gr}:100 \text{ mg}$$
$$1000 \text{ x} = 1500$$
$$x = {}^{1500}\!/_{1000}$$
$$x = 1\tfrac{1}{2} \text{ gr}$$

Solution 2:
$$1 \text{ gr}:65 \text{ mg} = x \text{ gr}:100 \text{ mg}$$
$$65 \text{ x} = 100$$
$$x = 1{}^{35}\!/_{65} \text{ gr}$$

Solution 3:
$$1 \text{ gr}:60 \text{ mg} - x \text{ gr}:100 \text{ mg}$$
$$60 \text{ x} = 100$$
$$x = 1\tfrac{2}{3} \text{ gr}$$

Solution 4:
$$1 \text{ gr}:64 \text{ mg} = x \text{ gr}:100 \text{ mg}$$
$$64 \text{ x} = 100$$
$$x = 1{}^{9}\!/_{16} \text{ gr}$$

Remembering the 10 percent margin of error rule, if the physician orders Nembutal 100 mg, no more than 110 mg or no less than 90 mg should be administered. This margin of difference allows for variances in determined dosages that will result from the particular equivalent values used. For example, Nembutal may be available in capsules containing gr ¾ and gr 1½. If gr 1 = 60 mg, then 1½ = 90 mg and 1 tablet labeled "gr 1½" may safely be given. If gr i = 64 mg, then gr iss (1½) = 96 mg and 1 tablet labeled "gr 1½" may be given. If gr i = 65 mg, then gr iss = 97.5 mg and 1 tablet labeled "gr 1½" may be given. This and most problems can be solved many different ways, giving slightly different but accurate answers.

Problem 4: 1 mg = ? gr

Solution 1:
$$15 \text{ gr}:1000 \text{ mg} = x \text{ gr}:1 \text{ mg}$$
$$1000 \text{ x} = 15$$
$$x = {}^{15}\!/_{1000}$$
$$x = {}^{3}\!/_{200} \text{ gr}$$

Solution 2:
$$16 \text{ gr}:1000 \text{ mg} = x \text{ gr}:1 \text{ mg}$$
$$1000 \text{ x} = 16$$
$$x = {}^{16}\!/_{1000}$$
$$x = {}^{4}\!/_{250}$$
$$x = {}^{2}\!/_{125} \text{ gr}$$

Problem 5: 1 dram (dr) = ? mL

Solution 1:
$$8 \text{ dr}:(1 \text{ oz}) \ 32 \text{ mL} = 1 \text{ dr}:x \text{ mL}$$
$$8 \text{ x} = 32$$
$$x = 4 \text{ mL}$$

Solution 2:
$$8 \text{ dr}:(1 \text{ oz}) \ 30 \text{ mL} = 1 \text{ dr}:x \text{ mL}$$
$$8 \text{ x} = 30$$
$$x = 3\tfrac{3}{4} \text{ mL}$$

It is suggested that the equivalents 1 teaspoon (tsp) equals 5 mL and 1 dr equals 4 mL be used when calculating dosages.

Problem 6: 1 tablespoon (Tbsp) = ? mL

Solution 1:   2 Tbsp:(1 oz) 30 mL = 1 Tbsp:x mL
$$2\ x = 20$$
$$x = 15\ mL$$

Solution 2:   2 Tbsp:(1 oz) 32 mL = 1 Tbsp:x mL
$$2\ x = 32$$
$$x = 16\ mL$$

Problem 7: 1 Tbsp = ? dr

Solution: (1 oz) 32 mL:8 dr = 16 mL:x dr
$$32\ x = 128$$
$$x = 4\ dr$$

If the number of milliliters in a tablespoon is not known, first determine this as shown in Problem 6.

Problem 8: 20 pounds (lb) = ? kilograms (kg)

Solution: 2.2 lb:1 kg = 20 lb:x kg
$$2.2x = 20$$
$$x = 9.09\ or\ 9.1\ kg$$

Practice Problems

Answers can be found in Appendix C, pp. 247–248.

Problem	Answer
1. ¾ gr = ? mg	
2. 0.3 g = ? gr	

Problem	Answer

3. 0.6 g = ? mg

4. 0.2 mg = ? gr

5. 750 mg = ? g

6. 0.005 gr = ? mg

7. 7½ gr = ? g

Problem	**Answer**

8. 2 fluid (fl) dr = ? mL

9. 1½ gr = ? g

10. 5 gr = ? mg

11. 1 Tbsp = ? mL

12. 0.03 g = ? mg

Problem	**Answer**

13. 130 lb = ? kg

14. 2 tsp = ? mL

15. 2 fl dr = ? mL

16. 20 mL = ? fl dr

17. 100 mg = ? gr

Problem	**Answer**

18. 10 gr = ? g

19. $\frac{1}{150}$ gr = ? mg

20. 7½ gr = ? mg

21. 0.01 mg = ? gr

22. $\frac{1}{60}$ gr = ? mg

Problem	**Answer**

23. 50 mg = ? gr

24. 1 mg = ? gr

25. 1/200 gr – ? mg

26. 0.1 g = ? gr

27. 0.3 g = ? gr

Problem	Answer

28. 5 gr = ? g

29. $\frac{1}{100}$ gr = ? g

30. 0.3 g = ? mg

31. 15 mL = ? fl dr

32. 1.5 g = ? mg

Problem	Answer

33. 2 Tbsp = ? mL

34. 0.01 g = ? mg

35. 20 mL = ? Tbsp

36. 500 mg = ? g

37. 6 kg = ? lb

Problem	**Answer**

38. 0.005 g = ? mg

39. 1½ glasses = ? mL

40. 150 mg = ? g

41. 7 lb = ? kg

42. ⅓ glass = ? mL

Problem	**Answer**

43. 55 kg = ? lb

44. 15 mL = ? teaspoons (tsp)

45. 180 lb = ? kg

46. 5000 g = ? lb

47. 2500 g = ? kg

Problem	**Answer**

48. 1800 g = ? lb

49. 1350 g = ? kg

50. 12 ounces (oz) = ? mL

CHAPTER 3

Nonparenteral Drugs

OBJECTIVES

At the end of this chapter, the student should be able to calculate accurately:
- Oral dosages using:
  - tablets and capsules
  - drugs in solution
- The preparation of oral and topical solutions using:
  - tablets, powders, and crystals
  - stock solutions

PART 10 • Oral Dosages

TABLETS AND CAPSULES

A general rule for administering ordered dosages of oral medications is that only scored tablets can be divided accurately. Examples of scored tablets can be seen in Figure 3–1. Usually one gives the ordered dosage using as few tablets as possible.

Enteric-coated tablets and capsules containing powders or timed-release pellets cannot be divided accurately. Therefore, it is necessary to look for capsules or enteric-coated tablets of the desired dosage or a dosage that falls within the 10 percent margin of error explained in Chapter 2.

Rarely does a physician order a drug in capsule or tablet form that is not available in the dosage ordered. The most frequent use of a fraction of a tablet occurs in the home when giving medications to a child using the available adult dosage tablet.

All tablets should be considered as unscored tablets unless otherwise indicated. All examples and practice problems involve the calculation of dosages for adults, except in Chapters 4, 5, and 6, which include children's dosages.

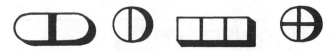

FIGURE 3–1 • Scored tablets.

Before discussing the calculation of oral tablet and capsule doses, it should be noted that this process occasionally is not necessary. The physician may order the exact number of tablets or capsules to be given. The practitioner may safely administer the number of tablets or capsules ordered *if* they are *certain* that the drug is available in one dosage only. For example, "clofibrate 1 capsule four times a day (qid)" could be administered safely, because clofibrate comes in 500 mg capsules only. However, by contrast, an order for "chlorpromazine 1 tablet three times a day (tid)" cannot be carried out safely because chlorpromazine is available in 10, 25, 50, 100, and 200 mg tablets.

Example Problems

Problem 1: ORDERED: Phenobarbital 60 mg PO bid
AVAILABLE: Phenobarbital 30 mg tablets

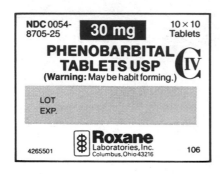

FIGURE 3–2 • Phenobarbital (Courtesy of Roxane Laboratories, Inc.).

Solution: FORMULA B

KNOWN AMOUNTS   UNKNOWN AMOUNTS
(AVAILABLE FOR USE)   (ORDERED)   (NEEDED)
dosage : amount = dosage : amount
30 mg : 1 tablet = 60 mg : x tablet(s)
$$30x = 60$$
$$x = {}^{60}\!/_{30}$$
$$x = 2 \text{ tablets}$$

Answer: Administer two phenobarbital tablets 30 mg each orally twice a day.

Whenever the available medication is labeled in the same unit of measure as the physician's order, only Formula B is needed to solve the problem, as in the previous example. Both Formula A and Formula B are needed to solve problems in which the available and ordered units of measure differ, as illustrated farther on. In such instances, note that one may convert the ordered dosage to the same unit of measure as the tablet available as illustrated in Problem 2, or one may convert the unit of measure of the tablet available to the same unit of measure as the ordered dosage as is illustrated in Problem 3.

Problem 2: ORDERED: Ferrous sulfate 5 gr PO bid
AVAILABLE: Ferrous sulfate 300 mg

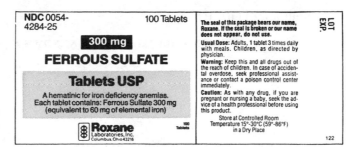

FIGURE 3–3 • Ferrous sulfate (Courtesy of Roxane Laboratories, Inc.).

Solution: FORMULA A

KNOWN EQUIVALENTS   UNKNOWN EQUIVALENTS

$$15 \text{ gr} : 1000 \text{ mg} = 5 \text{ gr} : x \text{ mg}$$
$$15x = 5000$$
$$x = {}^{5000}/_{15}$$
$$x = 333.3 \text{ mg}$$

Therefore, 5 gr ordered equals 333 mg.

Solution: FORMULA B

KNOWN AMOUNTS   UNKNOWN AMOUNTS
(AVAILABLE FOR USE)   (ORDERED)   (NEEDED)

$$300 \text{ mg} : 1 \text{ tablet} = 333 \text{ mg} : x \text{ tablet(s)}$$
$$300x = 333$$
$$x = {}^{333}/_{300}$$
$$x = 1.1 \text{ tablets}$$

Answer: Administer 1 ferrous sulfate tablet orally twice a day.

If the equivalent 1 gr:60 had been used in the previous example, then 5 gr would equal 300 mg. Actually, whenever a tablet is labeled 300 mg, 325 mg, 330 mg, 0.3 g, or 0.33 g, one may assume that this equals 5 gr. Conversely, one may assume that a tablet labeled 5 gr equals 300 mg or 325 mg, 330 mg, 0.3 g, or 0.33 g. Likewise, 10 gr equals 600 mg, 650 mg, 660 mg, 0.6 g, or 0.66 g. Remembering this can eliminate much difficulty when doing dosage problems.

Problem 3: ORDERED: Phenobarbital 1½ gr PO hs prn
AVAILABLE: Phenobarbital 100 mg tablets

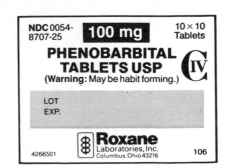

FIGURE 3–4 • Phenobarbital (Courtesy of Roxane Laboratories, Inc.).

Solution: FORMULA A

KNOWN EQUIVALENTS   UNKNOWN EQUIVALENTS

$$60 \text{ mg} : 1 \text{ gr} = 100 \text{ mg} : x \text{ gr}$$
$$60x = 100$$
$$x = {}^{100}\!/_{60}$$
$$x = 1.67 \text{ gr}$$

or

$$64 \text{ mg} : 1 \text{ gr} = 100 \text{ mg} : x \text{ gr}$$
$$64x = 100$$
$$x = {}^{100}\!/_{64}$$
$$x = 1.56 \text{ gr}$$

or

$$1000 \text{ mg} : 15 \text{ gr} = 100 \text{ mg} : x \text{ gr}$$
$$1000x = 1500$$
$$x = {}^{1500}\!/_{1000}$$
$$x = 1\tfrac{1}{2} \text{ gr}$$

Solution: FORMULA B

KNOWN AMOUNTS   UNKNOWN AMOUNTS
(AVAILABLE FOR USE)   (ORDERED)   (NEEDED)

$$\text{dosage} : \text{amount} = \text{dosage} : \text{amount}$$
$$1\tfrac{1}{2} \text{ gr} : 1 \text{ tablet} = 1\tfrac{1}{2} \text{ gr} : x \text{ tablet(s)}$$
$$1\tfrac{1}{2}x = 1\tfrac{1}{2}$$
$$x = \frac{1\tfrac{1}{2}}{1\tfrac{1}{2}}$$
$$x = 1 \text{ tablet}$$

Answer: Administer one phenobarbital 100 mg tablet orally at hour of sleep (bedtime) when required.

Problem 4: ORDERED: Gantrisin 7½ gr PO q4h
AVAILABLE: Sulfisoxazole (Gantrisin) 0.5 g tablets

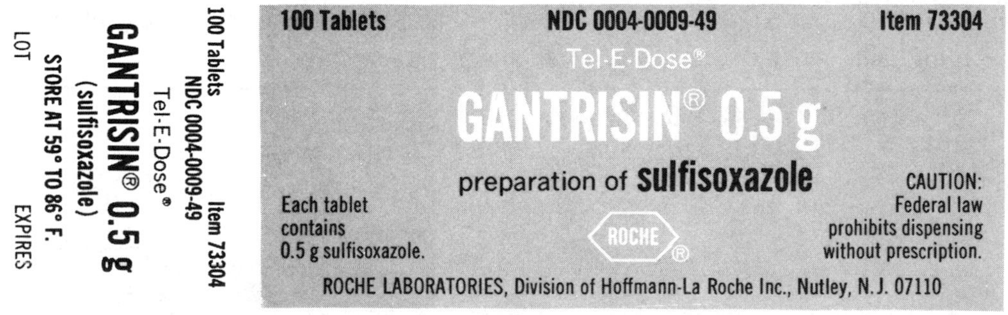

FIGURE 3–5 • Sulfisoxazole (Courtesy of Roche Laboratories).

Solution: FORMULA A

$$15 \text{ gr} : 1 \text{ g} = 7\tfrac{1}{2} \text{ gr} : x \text{ g}$$
$$15x = 7.5$$
$$x = {}^{7.5}\!/_{15}$$
$$x = 0.5 \text{ g}$$

Answer: Administer one sulfisoxazole 0.5 g tablet orally every 4 hours.

Problem 5: ORDERED: Digoxin $\frac{1}{120}$ gr PO qd
AVAILABLE: Digoxin (Lanoxin) scored tablets
0.25 mg

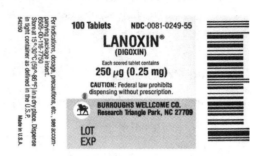

FIGURE 3–6 • Digoxin (Courtesy of Burroughs Wellcome Co.).

Solution: FORMULA A

$$1 \text{ mg} : \frac{1}{60} \text{ gr} = x \text{ mg} : \frac{1}{120} \text{ gr}$$
$$\frac{1}{60}x = \frac{1}{120}$$
$$x = \frac{1}{120} \div \frac{1}{60}$$
$$x = \frac{1}{120} \times \frac{60}{1}$$
$$x = \frac{60}{120} = \frac{1}{2}$$
$$x = 0.5 \text{ mg}$$

Solution: FORMULA B

$$0.25 \text{ mg} : 1 \text{ tablet} = 0.5 \text{ mg} : x \text{ tablet(s)}$$
$$0.25x = 0.5$$
$$x = 0.5 \div 0.25$$
$$x = 2 \text{ tablets}$$

Answer: Administer two Lanoxin tablets 0.25 mg each orally each day.

Problem 6: ORDERED: Dipyridamole 0.05 g PO tid ac
AVAILABLE: Dipyridamole 25 mg tablets

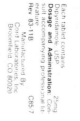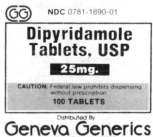

FIGURE 3–7 • Dipyridamole (Courtesy of Geneva Generics).

Solution: FORMULA A

$$1 \text{ g} : 1000 \text{ mg} = 0.05 \text{ g} : x \text{ mg}$$
$$1x = 50$$
$$x = 50 \text{ mg}$$

Solution: FORMULA B

$$25 \text{ mg} : 1 \text{ tablet} = 50 \text{ mg} : x \text{ tablet(s)}$$
$$25x = 50$$
$$x = 2 \text{ tablets}$$

Answer: Administer two dipyridamole tablets 25 mg each orally three times a day before meals.

Practice Problems

Answers can be found in Appendix C, pp. 248–249.

Problem	Answer

1. ORDERED: Diazepam gr ⅙ PO bid
   AVAILABLE: Diazepam 10 mg tablets

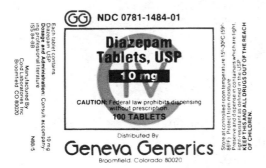

FIGURE 3–8 • Diazepam (Courtesy of Geneva Generics).

2. ORDERED: Erythromycin 0.5 g PO q6h
   AVAILABLE: Erythromycin stearate 250 mg tablets

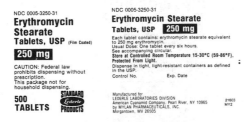

FIGURE 3–9 • Erythromycin stearate (Courtesy of Lederle Laboratories).

3. ORDERED: Neomycin 1 g and erythromycin 1 g PO at 1300, 1400, and 2100 h today

Problem	**Answer**

AVAILABLE: Neomycin sulfate
0.5 g tablets and erythromycin
stearate 500 mg tablets

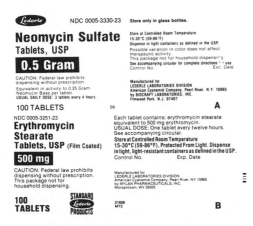

FIGURE 3–10 • Neomycin sulfate and erythromycin stearate (Courtesy of Lederle Laboratories).

4. ORDERED: Cortone 12.5 mg PO
qid
AVAILABLE: Cortisone acetate
(Cortone) 25 mg scored tablets

MSD   NDC 0006-0219-68

100 TABLETS

CORTONE® Acetate

(CORTISONE ACETATE, MSD)

25 mg

MERCK SHARP & DOHME
DIV OF MERCK & CO., INC., WEST POINT, PA 19486, USA

FIGURE 3–11 • Cortisone acetate (Courtesy
of Merck Sharp & Dohme).

5. ORDERED: Cortisone 0.05 g PO
qid
AVAILABLE: Cortisone acetate
(Cortone) 25 mg scored tablets

USUAL ADULT DOSAGE.
See accompanying circular.

This is a bulk package and
not intended for dispensing.

Dispense in a well closed container

CAUTION: Federal (USA) law prohibits dispensing without prescription

7570521

100 : No 7063

MSD   NDC 0006-0219-68

100 TABLETS

CORTONE® Acetate

(CORTISONE ACETATE, MSD)

25 mg

MERCK SHARP & DOHME
DIV OF MERCK & CO., INC., WEST POINT, PA 19486, USA

FIGURE 3–12 • Cortisone acetate (Courtesy
of Merck Sharp & Dohme).

Problem	**Answer**

6. Flurazepam ¼ gr PO at 2100 h prn
   and repeat one time, if needed
   AVAILABLE: Flurazepam
   hydrochloride (Flurazepam)
   15 mg capsules

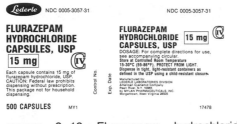

FIGURE 3–13 • Flurazepam hydrochloride (Courtesy of Lederle Laboratories).

7. ORDERED: Phenergan 0.025 g PO
   bid
   AVAILABLE: Promethazine
   hydrochloride (Phenergan)
   12.5 mg tablets

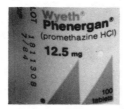

FIGURE 3–14 • Promethazine hydrochloride (From Wyeth Laboratories, Inc. with permission).

8. ORDERED: Digoxin 0.75 mg PO
   stat
   AVAILABLE: Digoxin (Lanoxin)
   500 mcg (0.5 mg) scored
   tablets

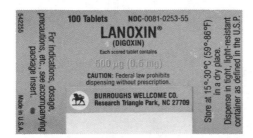

FIGURE 3–15 • Digoxin (Courtesy of Burroughs Wellcome Co.).

Problem	**Answer**

9. ORDERED: Demerol 0.1 g PO q4h
   prn for pain
   AVAILABLE: Meperidine
   hydrochloride (Demerol) 100
   mg tablets

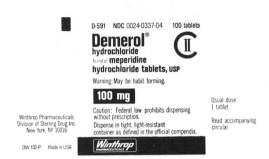

FIGURE   3–16 • Meperidine   hydrochloride
(Courtesy of Winthrop Pharmaceuticals).

10. ORDERED: Flurazepam ½ gr PO
    hs
    AVAILABLE: Flurazepam
    hydrochloride (Flurazepam)
    30 mg capsules

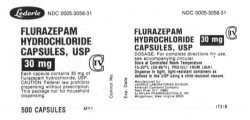

FIGURE   3–17 • Flurazepam   hydrochloride
(Courtesy of Lederle Laboratories).

11. ORDERED: Demerol 0.1 g PO q3h
    prn for pain
    AVAILABLE: Meperidine
    hydrochloride (Demerol) 50
    mg tablets

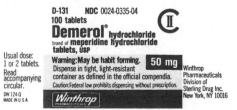

FIGURE   3–18 • Meperidine   hydrochloride
(Courtesy of Winthrop Pharmaceuticals).

Problem	Answer

12. ORDERED: Lanoxin ½₂₅₀ gr PO
    q8h today
    AVAILABLE: Digoxin (Lanoxin)
    250 mcg (0.25 mg) scored
    tablets

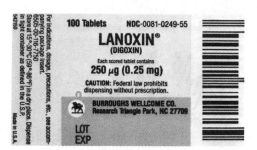

FIGURE 3–19 • Digoxin (Courtesy of Burroughs Wellcome Co.).

13. ORDERED: Cortone 75 mg PO
    stat, initial dose
    AVAILABLE: Cortisone acetate
    (Cortone) 25 mg scored tablets

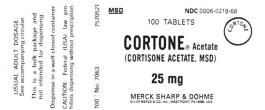

FIGURE 3–20 • Cortisone acetate (Courtesy of Merck Sharp & Dohme).

14. ORDERED: Furosemide 80 mg PO
    q6h today only (four doses)
    AVAILABLE: Furosemide 20 mg
    tablets

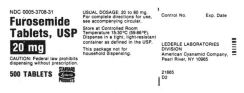

FIGURE 3–21 • Furosemide (Courtesy of Lederle Laboratories).

Problem	**Answer**

15. ORDERED: Phenobarbital ½ gr
    PO qid
    AVAILABLE: Phenobarbital 15
    mg tablets

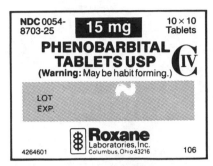

FIGURE 3–22 • Phenobarbital (Courtesy of Roxane Laboratories, Inc.).

16. ORDERED: Nembutal 1½ gr PO
    at 2100 h
    AVAILABLE: Pentobarbital
    sodium (Nembutal) 50 mg
    tablets

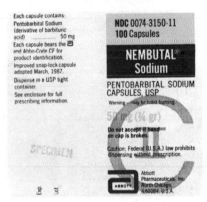

FIGURE 3–23 • Pentobarbital sodium (Courtesy of Abbott Laboratories).

17. ORDERED: Erythromycin 500 mg
    PO tid
    AVAILABLE: Erythromycin
    stearate 250 mg tablets

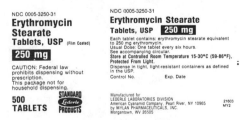

FIGURE 3–24 • Erythromycin stearate (Courtesy of Lederle Laboratories).

Problem	**Answer**

18. ORDERED: Flurazepam HCl ½ gr
    PO bid
    AVAILABLE: Flurazepam
    hydrochloride 30 mg capsules

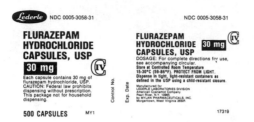

FIGURE 3–25 • Flurazepam hydrochloride (Courtesy of Lederle Laboratories).

19. ORDERED: Gantrisin 500 mg PO
    qid
    AVAILABLE: Sulfisoxazole
    (Gantrisin) 0.5 g tablets

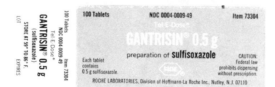

FIGURE 3–26 • Sulfisoxazole (Courtesy of Roche Laboratories).

20. ORDERED: Ferrous sulfate 0.3 g
    PO qid
    AVAILABLE: Ferrous sulfate 300
    mg tablets

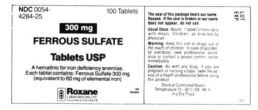

FIGURE 3–27 • Ferrous sulfate (Courtesy of Roxane Laboratories, Inc.).

21. ORDERED: Neomycin 1000 mg
    PO q4h for 24 h (total of six
    doses)
    AVAILABLE: Neomycin sulfate
    0.5 g

Problem   **Answer**

NEOMYCIN SULFATE
TABLETS, USP
0.5 Gram
(Equivalent to 0.35 Gram of Neomycin Base)

FIGURE 3–28 • Neomycin sulfate (Courtesy of Lederle Laboratories).

22. ORDERED: Lanoxin 0.25 mg PO
      daily
    AVAILABLE: Digoxin (Lanoxin)
      250 mcg scored tablets

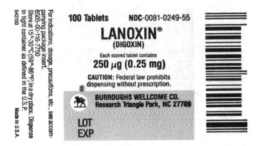

FIGURE 3–29 • Digoxin (Courtesy of Burroughs Wellcome Co.).

23. ORDERED: Demerol 0.05 g PO
      q4h prn pain
    AVAILABLE: Meperidine
      hydrochloride (Demerol) 100
      mg tablets

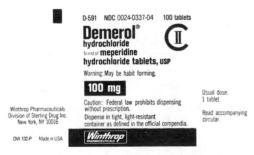

FIGURE 3–30 • Meperidine hydrochloride (Courtesy of Winthrop Pharmaceuticals).

24. ORDERED: Dipyridamole 0.025 g
      PO tid ac
    AVAILABLE: Dipyridamole 25
      mg tablets

Problem	Answer

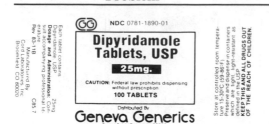

FIGURE 3–31 • Dipyridamole (Courtesy of Geneva Generics).

DRUGS IN SOLUTION

Drugs Not Requiring Calculations

Some drugs are available in one strength only. They usually do not have a specific weight measure of drug in a specified volume of solvent. With these drugs, the physician orders the exact volume amount to be given. No calculation is necessary to determine the amount of the drug to be given. The volume ordered becomes the amount to be administered. Some examples of such orders are as follows:

> Alurate elixir ℥ ÷ PO q3–4h prn
> Milk of magnesia ℥ ÷ stat
> Terpin hydrate elixir 5 mL q4h prn for cough
> Gelusil 30 mL tid ac and hs
> Robitussin 5 cc q2h prn for cough
> 10% potassium chloride liquid 15 mL tid
> Paregoric 5 mL stat
> Donnatal elixir 5 cc tid ac and hs
> Parapectolin 5 cc prn for diarrhea

One-ounce receptacles (Fig. 3–32) used for administering drugs orally vary, but most are marked in drams and milliliters (or cc) and many also include teaspoon and tablespoon measurements. Therefore, relatively large amounts can be measured quite accurately in 1-ounce (oz) containers.

Other more accurate means should be used to measure less than 5 mL and smaller units of measure such as minims and drops. Figure 3–33 shows an oral syringe used to

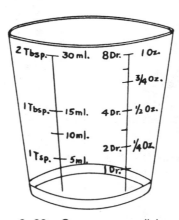

FIGURE 3–32 • One ounce medicine cup.

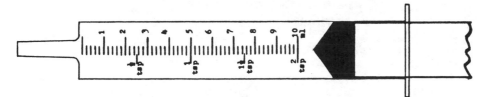

FIGURE 3–33 • Oral syringe.

measure from 0.2 mL to 10 mL of solution. A tuberculin syringe can be used to measure up to 16 minims or hundredths of a milliliter (Fig. 4–1, page 94).

A drop is an approximate household unit of measurement; a minim is an accurate apothecaries' unit of measurement. Therefore, one may safely substitute minims for drops, but one should never measure a dosage in drops when minims are ordered. Minim pipettes or syringes may be used to measure minims. Medicine droppers are used to measure drops. The size of drops varies considerably depending upon the viscosity and temperature of the solution, the size of the opening in the dropper, the force with which the solution is expelled, and the angle at which the dropper is held. Holding the dropper at a 45-degree angle is suggested when measuring drugs.

Some liquid drugs come with a special graduated dropper attached to the lid of the bottle, as illustrated in Figure 3–34. These are graduated to be used with the specific drug in the bottle to which they are attached.

Drugs Requiring Calculations

When physicians order oral preparations of drugs in solution, they frequently order a number of milligrams, grams, or other units of weight measures. Health-care personnel must then convert these to drams, ounces, milliliters, or other units of volume measure in order to administer the prescribed dosage.

When practitioners must use weight to fluid volume measurements to solve dosage or solution problems, the equivalents of 1 g equals 1 mL and 1 gr equals 1 m are those most frequently used.

Labels on drugs in solution may indicate a certain weight measure in a particular volume measure—for example, 500 mg per mL or 10 gr in 1 dr. Labels of these drugs also may merely state a percentage (1.0%) or a ratio (1:200) strength of the solutions as illustrated by Figure 3–35.

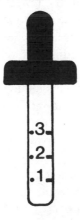

FIGURE 3–34 • Calibrated medicine dropper.

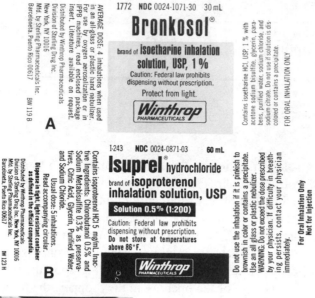

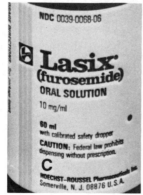

FIGURE 3–35 • Three different labels. **(A)** Isoetharine (Courtesy of Winthrop Pharmaceuticals). **(B)** Isoproterenol (Courtesy of Winthrop Pharmaceuticals). **(C)** Furosemide (Courtesy of Hoechst-Roussel Pharmaceuticals, Inc.).

Whenever the strength of a drug that is available in solution is stated as a ratio or as a percentage strength, the parts are equal parts. A 5% solution, therefore, may be said to contain 5 g in every 100 mL because 1 g = 1 mL. It may also be said to contain 5 gr in every 100 m because 1 gr = 1 m. A 1:1000 solution contains 1 gr in every 1000 m, 1 g in every 1000 mL, 1000 mg in every 1000 mL, or 1 mg in every 1 mL. One gram of a drug usually does not exactly equal 1 mL, but when administering drugs in solution form, we can assume this equality because the pharmacist or pharmaceutical company has weighed, not measured, the drug.

It does not matter how much of the drug one says is available for administration in the first and second terms of the proportion when calculating the dosage. It is only the strength of the solution available for administration that is important. After determining how much of the solution is needed in order to give the desired dosage, one can determine whether the drug container contains enough solution for the ordered dosage.

Units of measure other than those found in the metric, apothecaries', or household systems may be used to indicate the quantity of a drug either in oral or parenteral solution. Units, abbreviated U, and milliequivalents, abbreviated mEq, are the most commonly used. Occasionally such units of measure are used for drugs in tablet or capsule form. Physicians order a quantity of milliequivalents or units. Labels on the drugs indicate the number of milliequivalents or units in a particular volume or capacity measure (e.g., 400,000 U per mL or 20 mEq per 15 mL).

A milliequivalent, which is equal to one thousandth of an equivalent, refers to the number of ionic charges of an element or a compound. It is a measure of the chemical combining power of a substance. Potassium chloride (KCl) is an example of a drug ordered in milliequivalents.

Measuring drugs in units means something a little different for every drug measured this way. One United States Pharmacopeia (USP) insulin unit promotes the metabolism of about 1.5 g of dextrose. A penicillin unit is the equivalent of the antibiotic activity of 0.6 mcg of USP Penicillin Sodium Reference Standard. One milligram of this kind of penicillin equals 1667 units. Other kinds of penicillin have different milligrams to units equivalents. For example, 1 mg of benzathine penicillin equals 1211 USP units.

Example Problems

Problem 1: ORDERED: Ceclor 0.4 g per gastric tube q8h
AVAILABLE: Cefaclor (Ceclor) oral suspension 250 mg/5 mL

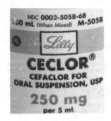

FIGURE 3–36 • Cefaclor (Courtesy of Eli Lilly & Co.).

Solution: FORMULA A

KNOWN EQUIVALENTS   UNKNOWN EQUIVALENTS
$$1000 \text{ mg}:1 \text{ g} = x \text{ mg}:0.4 \text{ g}$$
$$1x = 1000 \times 0.4$$
$$x = 400 \text{ mg}$$

Solution: FORMULA B

KNOWN AMOUNTS   UNKNOWN AMOUNTS
(AVAILABLE FOR USE)   (ORDERED)   (NEEDED)
$$\text{dosage}:\text{amount} = \text{dosage}:\text{amount}$$
$$250 \text{ mg}:5 \text{ mL} = 400 \text{ mg}:x \text{ mL}$$
$$250x = 2000$$
$$x = {}^{2000}\!/_{240}$$
$$x = 8 \text{ mL}$$

Answer: Add 90 mL water as directed to powder, shake well, and give 8 mL per gastric tube every 8 hours.

Problem 2: ORDERED: Dextrose 2.5 g PO tid today
AVAILABLE: Dextrose 5% solution in a 250 mL bag

Solution:
$$5 \text{ g}:100 \text{ mL} = 2.5 \text{ g}:x \text{ mL}$$
$$5x = 250$$
$$x = 50 \text{ mL}$$

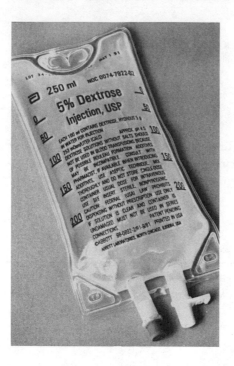

FIGURE 3–37 • Dextrose 5% (Courtesy of Abbott Laboratories).

Answer: Administer 50 mL of 5% dextrose solution orally three times today.

Problem 3: ORDERED: Isotonic sodium chloride (NaCl) 1.0 g PO q6h today
AVAILABLE: 0.9% sodium chloride solution in a 250 mL bag

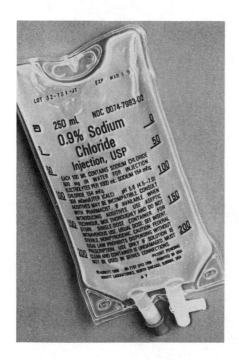

FIGURE 3–38 • Isotonic sodium chloride (Courtesy of Abbott Laboratories).

Solution:

$$0.9 \text{ g}:100 \text{ mL} = 1 \text{ g}:x \text{ mL}$$
$$0.9x = 100$$
$$x = 100 \div \frac{9}{10}$$

$$x = {}^{100}\!/_1 \times {}^{10}\!/_9$$
$$x = {}^{1000}\!/_9$$
$$x = 111\tfrac{1}{9}\ \text{mL}$$

Answer: Administer approximately 111⅑ mL isotonic NaCl solution by mouth every 6 hours today.

Problem 4: ORDERED: Lasix 0.05 g PO bid

AVAILABLE: Furosemide (Lasix) oral solution 10 mg/mL in 120 mL bottles

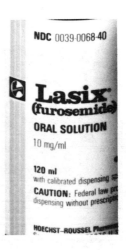

FIGURE 3–39 • Furosemide (Courtesy of Hoechst-Roussel Pharmaceuticals, Inc.).

Solution: FORMULA A

$$1\ \text{g}:1000\ \text{mg} = 0.05\ \text{g}:x\ \text{mg}$$
$$1x = 1000 \times 0.05$$
$$1x = 50$$
$$x = 50\ \text{mg}$$

Solution: FORMULA B

$$10\ \text{mg}:1\ \text{mL} = 50\ \text{mg}:x\ \text{mL}$$
$$10x = 50$$
$$x = 5\ \text{mL}$$

Answer: Pour 5 mL of furosemide oral solution from a bottle labeled furosemide oral solution 10 mg/mL and administer by mouth twice a day.

Problem 5: ORDERED: Diphenhydramine hydrochloride elixir 20 mg PO q6h

AVAILABLE: Diphenhydramine hydrochloride elixir 25 mg/10 mL

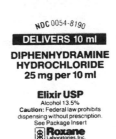

FIGURE 3–40 • Diphenhydramine hydrochloride (Courtesy of Roxane Laboratories, Inc.).

Solution:
$$25 \text{ mg}:10 \text{ mL} = 20 \text{ mg}:x \text{ mL}$$
$$25x = 200$$
$$x = {}^{200}\!/_{25}$$
$$x = 8 \text{ mL}$$

Answer: Administer 8 mL diphenhydramine hydrochloride elixir by mouth every 6 hours.

Problem 6: ORDERED: Pen-Vee K 500,000 U PO q4h

AVAILABLE: Penicillin V potassium (Pen-Vee K) 250 mg (400,000 U)/5 mL in 100 mL bottle

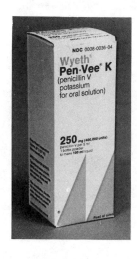

FIGURE 3–41 • Penicillin V potassium (From Wyeth Laboratories, Inc. with permission).

Solution:
$$400,000 \text{ U}:5 \text{ mL} = 500,000 \text{ U}:x \text{ mL}$$
$$400,000x = 2,500,000$$
$$x = 6.25 \text{ mL}$$

Answer: Administer 6.25 mL penicillin V potassium labeled 400,000 U in 5 mL by mouth every 4 hours.

Practice Problems

Answers can be found in Appendix C, pp. 249–250.

Problem	Answer

1. ORDERED: Paregoric ℥i stat
   AVAILABLE: Paregoric 5 mL

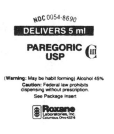

FIGURE 3–42 • Paregoric (Courtesy of Roxane Laboratories, Inc.).

Problem	Answer

2. ORDERED: Penicillin VK 0.5 g
PO q6h
AVAILABLE: Penicillin V
potassium (Pen-Vee K) 125
mg/5mL

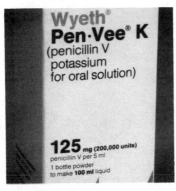

FIGURE 3–43 • Penicillin V potassium (From Wyeth Laboratories, Inc. with permission).

3. ORDERED: Amicar 1 g q3h
AVAILABLE: Aminocaproic acid
(Amicar) syrup 25% in a 16
oz bottle

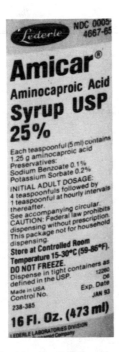

FIGURE 3–44 • Aminocaproic acid (From Lederle Laboratories with permission).

4. ORDERED: Mycostatin oral
suspension 500,000 U tid

Problem	Answer

AVAILABLE: Nystatin
(Mycostatin) oral suspension
100,000 U/mL in 60 mL
bottle

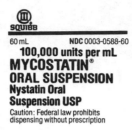

FIGURE 3–45 • Nystatin (Courtesy of E. R. Squibb & Sons, Inc.).

5. ORDERED: Phenobarbital elixir 15 mg PO tid
   AVAILABLE: Phenobarbital elixir 20 mg/5 mL

FIGURE 3–46 • Phenobarbital (Courtesy of Roxane Laboratories, Inc.).

6. ORDERED: Acetaminophen elixir (160 mg/5 mL) 2 tsp q4h prn
   AVAILABLE: Acetaminophen elixir 160 mg/5 mL in 120 mL bottle

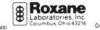

FIGURE 3–47 • Acetaminophen (Courtesy of Roxane Laboratories, Inc.).

Problem	Answer

7. ORDERED: Atarax syrup 15 mg
   PO qid
   AVAILABLE: Hydroxyzine
   hydrochloride (Atarax) syrup
   10 mg/5 mL

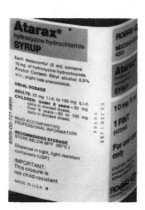

FIGURE 3–48 • Hydroxyzine hydrochloride
(From Roerig with permission).

8. ORDERED: Digoxin 0.4 mg PO
   qd
   AVAILABLE: Digoxin (Lanoxin)
   pediatric elixir 0.05 mg (50
   mcg)/mL in a 60 mL bottle

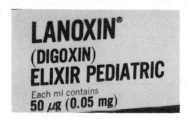

FIGURE 3–49 • Digoxin (From Burroughs
Wellcome Co. with permission).

9. ORDERED: Polymox suspension
   100 mg tid
   AVAILABLE: Amoxicillin
   (Polymox) oral suspension
   125 mg/5 mL in 80 mL bottle

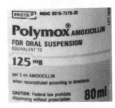

FIGURE 3–50 • Amoxicillin (From Bristol Laboratories with permission).

Problem	Answer

10. ORDERED: Phenergan with codeine
gr ⅙ q6h prn for cough
AVAILABLE: Promethazine
hydrochloride (Phenergan)
6.25 mg/5 mL and codeine
phosphate 10 mg/5 mL.
(Calculate using codeine dose,
since Phenergan dose does not
change.)

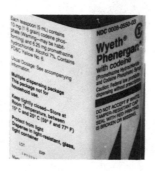

FIGURE 3–51 • Promethazine hydrochloride and codeine phosphate (From Wyeth Laboratories, Inc. with permission).

11. ORDERED: Amicar syrup 5 g stat,
then 1 g qh for 8 h
AVAILABLE: Aminocaproic acid
(Amicar) syrup 25% (250
mg/mL) in 16 oz bottles

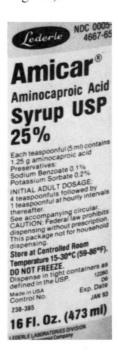

FIGURE 3–52 • Aminocaproic acid (From Lederle Laboratories with permission).

Problem	**Answer**

12. ORDERED: Kaon Elixir 12 mEq
     bid
     AVAILABLE: Potassium
     gluconate (Kaon Elixir) 20
     mEq/15 mL in 500 mL bottle

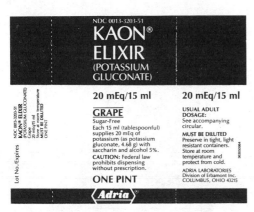

FIGURE 3–53 • Potassium gluconate (Courtesy of Adria Laboratories).

13. ORDERED: Butisol elixir 50 mg
     PO stat
     AVAILABLE: Butabarbital sodium
     elixir (Butisol) 30 mg/5 mL in
     1 pint (pt) bottle

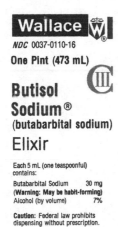

FIGURE 3–54 • Butabarbitol sodium (Courtesy of Wallace Laboratories).

14. ORDERED: Acetaminophen elixir
     240 mg PO for temperature
     over 102°F
     AVAILABLE: Acetaminophen
     elixir 160 mg/5 mL in 120 mL
     bottle

Problem	Answer

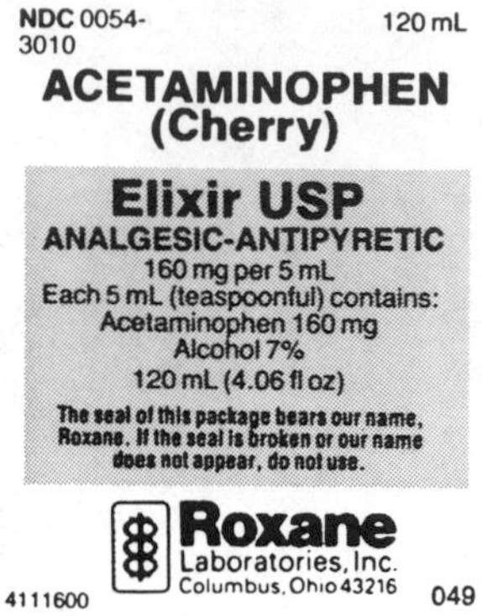

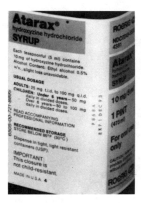

FIGURE 3–55 • Acetaminophen (Courtesy of Roxane Laboratories, Inc.).

15. ORDERED: Atarax syrup 40 mg
        PO stat
     AVAILABLE: Hydroxyzine
        hydrochloride syrup (Atarax)
        10 mg/5 mL in 1 pt bottle

FIGURE 3–56 • Hydroxyzine hydrochloride (From Roerig with permission).

16. ORDERED: Polymox suspension
        0.5 g PO stat, then qid
     AVAILABLE: Amoxicillin
        (Polymox) suspension 125
        mg/5 mL in 80 mL bottle

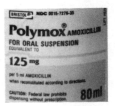

FIGURE 3–57 • Amoxicillin (From Bristol Laboratories with permission).

Problem	**Answer**

17. ORDERED: Amicar syrup 1 g PO
     qh prn, limit six doses
     AVAILABLE: Aminocaproic acid
     syrup (Amicar) 25% in 16 oz
     bottles

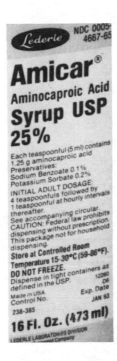

FIGURE 3–58 • Aminocaproic acid (From
Lederle Laboratories with permission).

18. ORDERED: Kaochlor 36 mEq
     daily in AM
     AVAILABLE: Potassium chloride
     (Kaochlor) 20 mEq/15 mL in
     500 mL bottle

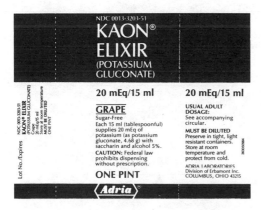

FIGURE 3–59 • Potassium chloride (Courtesy
of Adria Laboratories).

Problem	**Answer**

19. ORDERED: Atarax syrup 0.03 g
    PO qid
    AVAILABLE: Hydroxyzine
    hydrochloride syrup (Atarax)
    10 mg/5 mL

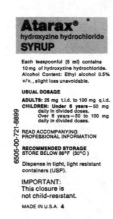

FIGURE 3–60 • Hydroxyzine hydrochloride (Courtesy of Roerig).

20. ORDERED: Gantrisin suspension
    100 mg PO qid
    AVAILABLE: Acetyl sulfisoxazole
    pediatric suspension
    (Gantrisin) 0.5 g/5 mL in 4 oz
    bottle

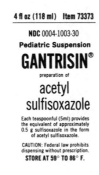

FIGURE 3–61 • Acetyl sulfisoxazole (Courtesy of Roche Laboratories).

PART 11 • Preparation of Oral and Topical Solutions

This section is included at the request of faculty members who have found that it helps the users understand the strength of drugs available in, or prepared in, solution form. Solutions used topically usually are available from stock supplies or are prepared by the pharmacy in the strength desired. Occasionally, however, in small hospitals or in community settings one may need to prepare solutions for hospital use or instruct patients how to prepare solutions for topical use in their homes. Also, one may need to know how to prepare solutions for oral use, such as a 1:3 solution of hydrogen peroxide as a mouthwash.

When preparing solutions for topical or oral use, one is changing the percentage or ratio strength of the drug to a weaker strength or to the strength ordered or desired for use. One or two variations of Formula B can be used to solve all types of solution problems, which include:

- Preparing solutions from tablets, powders, or crystals (always 100% strength)
- Preparing solutions from:
  - 100% strength stock solutions
  - less than 100% strength stock solutions

Although the substance (solutes) added to the solvent do increase the total volume slightly, the amount of total increase is too small to make any appreciable difference when preparing large amounts of solutions. For example, the displacement by the solute may be 0.5 mL or 2 mL when one is preparing 1000 mL of solution and one is using a 1 liter pitcher with a mark every 50 mL to measure the solvent. It is impossible to measure accurately enough to account for such small displacements. Therefore, the amount of displacement by the drug in an oral or topical solution is not taken into consideration when the drug used is in tablet, crystal, or powder form.

TABLETS, POWDERS, OR CRYSTALS

Occasionally one needs to prepare an oral solution from tablets as in Problem 1. Sometimes they may need to prepare children's doses from adult dosage tablets if the drug is not readily available in the pediatric liquid or tablet form and the tablet available cannot be divided accurately by breaking it. If the tablet is soluble in water, it can be crushed and dissolved in a specific amount of water. Then the ordered dosage can be accurately measured in a syringe (Problem 1, Solution 1).

Example Problems

Problem 1: ORDERED: Sudafed 10 mg PO q6h

AVAILABLE: Pseudoephedrine hydrochloride (Sudafed) 60 mg tablets

Solution 1: First, use Formula B to determine the fraction of the tablet that will be needed.

KNOWN AMOUNTS   UNKNOWN AMOUNTS

$$60 \text{ mg}:1 \text{ tablet} = 10 \text{ mg}:x \text{ tablet}$$
$$60x = 10$$
$$x = {}^{10}\!/_{60}$$
$$x = \frac{1}{6} \text{ tablet}$$

Answer: In this instance, the denominator can be interpreted as the total volume in which to dissolve the tablet (for example, 6 mL). The numerator can then be interpreted as the dose to be given (in this example, 1 mL).

Solution 2: One can arbitrarily choose the amount of solution in which to give the ordered dose of the drug. In this example, the practitioner chose to use 4 mL.

KNOWN AMOUNTS   UNKNOWN AMOUNTS
(TO BE PREPARED FOR USE)   (TO BE PREPARED FOR USE)
(STRENGTH TO BE PREPARED)   (TOTAL TO BE PREPARED)

$$\text{dosage}:\text{amount} = \text{dosage}:\text{amount}$$
$$10 \text{ mg}:4 \text{ mL} = 60 \text{ mg}:x \text{ mL}$$
$$10x = 240$$
$$x = {}^{240}\!/_{10}$$
$$x = 24 \text{ mL}$$

Answer: Therefore, if one wants to give 10 mg in 4 mL, dissolve 1 of the 60 mg Sudafed tablets in 24 mL of solution and give 4 mL orally every 6 hours.

Solution 3: Or, one can choose the amount of solution in which to dissolve the tablet. In this example, the practitioner chose to use 30 mL. A 1 oz medicine glass could be used.

KNOWN AMOUNTS   UNKNOWN AMOUNTS
(TO BE PREPARED FOR USE)   (TO BE PREPARED FOR USE)
(TOTAL TO BE PREPARED)   (STRENGTH TO BE PREPARED)

$$\text{dosage}:\text{amount} = \text{dosage}:\text{amount}$$
$$60 \text{ mg}:30 \text{ mL} = 10 \text{ mg}:x \text{ mL}$$
$$60x = 300$$
$$x = {}^{300}\!/_{60}$$
$$x = 5 \text{ mL}$$

Answer: Therefore, if one chooses to dissolve 1 of the 60 mg Sudafed tablets in 30 mL of water, do so, and give 5 mL orally every 6 hours.

Problem 2: ORDERED: 250 mL ½ isotonic saline PO qh × 4
AVAILABLE: Table salt and home cooking measures

It should be remembered that isotonic saline is a 0.9% strength solution and that 1 g = 1 mL. Because the oral solution is ordered for four doses (× 4), it would be easier to prepare all four doses at one time, or 1000 mL (4 × 250 mL).

Solution: FORMULA B

KNOWN AMOUNTS   UNKNOWN AMOUNTS
(TO BE PREPARED FOR USE)   (TO BE PREPARED FOR USE)
(STRENGTH TO BE PREPARED)   (TOTAL TO BE PREPARED)

$$\text{dosage} : \text{amount} = \text{dosage} : \text{amount}$$
$$0.45 \text{ g} : 100 \text{ mL} = x \text{ g} : 1000 \text{ mL}$$
$$100x = 450$$
$$x = {}^{450}\!/_{100}$$
$$x = 4.5 \text{ g}$$

Answer: Add 4.5 g (1 tsp) salt to 1 qt (1000 mL) of water if preparing the entire amount at one time, or ¼ tsp salt to a glass of water (250 mL) if preparing one dose at a time. Because of the heavy molecular weight of sodium chloride, 2 tsp of salt per quart of water may be used when preparing isotonic saline solutions (1 tsp per quart when preparing ½ isotonic saline solution).

In actual practice, the containers available for measurement of large volumes are calibrated for every 50 or 100 mL. Accurate measurement of the stock drug or solution to within a fraction of a milliliter or even to within a few milliliters is not possible when the calibration is this large. It may be necessary to measure the small amounts of solute (the medication) in a 1 oz container and to measure the solvent (the liquid) in another much larger container.

Problem 3: ORDERED: Warm saturated boric acid solution soaks to left foot 20 min stat (assume that one needs 1 gal of this solution)

AVAILABLE: Boric acid crystals

Solution: A 5% boric acid solution is a saturated one.

KNOWN AMOUNTS	UNKNOWN AMOUNTS
(TO BE PREPARED FOR USE)	(TO BE PREPARED FOR USE)
(STRENGTH TO BE PREPARED)	(TOTAL TO BE PREPARED)

$$\text{dosage} : \text{amount} = \text{dosage} : \text{amount}$$
$$5 \text{ g} : 100 \text{ mL} = x \text{ g (mL)} : 4000 \text{ mL}$$
$$100x = 20{,}000$$
$$x = {}^{20{,}000}\!/_{100}$$
$$x = 200 \text{ g (mL)}$$

Answer: Add 200 mL boric acid crystals to 1 gallon (gal) warm water and soak left foot in it for 20 minutes immediately.

Weighing 200 g of boric acid crystals would be more accurate than measuring 200 mL of the drug, but gram scales are usually not available in clinical areas or homes. When preparing solutions for topical use, attaining the exact ordered strength is not as important as when giving oral or parenteral dosages. Therefore, in this instance, one may safely substitute milliliters for grams when measuring powders or crystals.

Problem 4: ORDERED: NS enema prn (one decides to prepare 2 qt of this solution)

AVAILABLE: Table salt

Normal saline (NS) is a 5.8% strength solution. Normal saline solutions are rarely used because they are physiologically hypertonic rather than isotonic. Physiologically isotonic saline is a 0.9% strength solution. However, when dealing with drugs in solution and parenteral fluids, the abbreviation ''NS'' is used for normal saline and the strength intended is 0.9%, the strength of isotonic saline. When ordered by the physician, ½ NS would be 0.45% strength and ¼ NS would be 0.225% strength. (Available solutions of ¼ NS are labeled 0.2%.)

Solution:

KNOWN AMOUNTS   UNKNOWN AMOUNTS

$$\text{dosage}:\text{amount} = \text{dosage}:\text{amount}$$
$$0.9 \text{ g}:100 \text{ mL} = x \text{ g (mL)}:2000 \text{ mL}$$
$$100x = 1800$$
$$x = {}^{1800}/_{100}$$
$$x = 18 \text{ g (mL)}$$

Answer: Add 18 mL (4 tsp) of table salt to 2 quarts (qt) of tap water at the appropriate temperature.

STOCK SOLUTIONS

As stated earlier, occasionally one may need to solve problems involving the dilution of stock solutions to make weaker solutions. The strength of the solution to be prepared for use may be stated as a ratio such as 1:4 or as a percentage strength such as 2%. The strength of the stock solution available also may be expressed as a ratio (1:100) or as a percentage strength (1%).

Remember, to represent properly the strength of a percent solution, the number before the percent sign equals the number of grams of the drug in 100 mL of solution or the number of grains in 100 m of solution. For example, a 5% solution can be said to contain 5 g of drug in every 100 mL of solution, or a 5% solution can be said to contain 5 gr of drug in every 100 m of solution. To represent properly the strength of a ratio solution, a 1:1000 solution can be said to contain 1 g of drug in every 1000 mL of solution (1 g in 1000 mL = 1000 mg in 1000 mL = 1 mg in 1 mL) or 1 gr of drug in every 1000 m of solution.

Whereas the amount of displacement by a powder, tablet, or crystal solute placed in a large volume of solvent is not taken into consideration when calculating the amount of solute to use, one must consider the displacement made by the stronger solution used to make a weaker solution. For example, if 2000 mL of a 25% solution is to be made from a 100% solution, the amount of the 100% solution needed for the dilution must be considered as displacement. The 25% solution would be one-fourth as strong as the 100% solution. One would be preparing a 1:4 strength solution with one part or 500 mL of 100% solution plus three parts or 1500 mL of water to get the four total parts.

Example Problems

Problem 1: ORDERED: Dilute hydrogen peroxide to 1:4 and use it as a mouthwash qid (one needs 1 oz for each treatment)
AVAILABLE: Hydrogen peroxide (3%)

Solution:

KNOWN AMOUNTS   UNKNOWN AMOUNTS
(TO BE PREPARED FOR USE)   (TO BE PREPARED FOR USE)
(STRENGTH TO BE PREPARED)   (TOTAL TO BE PREPARED)

$$\text{dosage}:\text{amount} = \text{dosage}:\text{amount}$$
$$1:4 = x \text{ mL}:32 \text{ mL}$$
$$4x = 32$$
$$x = 3\tfrac{2}{4}$$
$$x = 8 \text{ mL}$$

Answer: Use 8 mL of 3% hydrogen peroxide and 24 mL water to get a total volume of 32 mL (one must account for the volume of the solution that is used in the dilution).

There are 20% hydrogen peroxide preparations but these are not for medicinal use. The 3% hydrogen peroxide is rarely used as a mouthwash without further dilution to 1:3 or 1:4 strength.

Problem 2: ORDERED: Hydrogen peroxide 1:3 as a mouthwash tid (one needs 2 oz for each treatment)
AVAILABLE: Hydrogen peroxide (3%)

Solution:

$$1:3 = x \text{ mL} : 60 \text{ mL}$$
$$3x = 60$$
$$x = {}^{60}\!/_3$$
$$x = 20 \text{ mL}$$

Answer: Use 20 mL of 3% hydrogen peroxide and 40 mL of water for each treatment.

When determining how to prepare solutions from stock solutions of less than 100% strength, two variations of Formula B must be used. The first step is to determine the amount of drug needed to prepare the desired strength and amount of solution. The second step is to determine the amount of stock solution needed in order to obtain this amount of drug. Examples follow:

Problem 3: ORDERED: 30% alcohol cooling sponge stat (assume one needs 2 qt of solution)
AVAILABLE: 70% isopropyl alcohol

Solution: Step 1. Amount of drug needed

KNOWN AMOUNTS   **UNKNOWN AMOUNTS**
(TO BE PREPARED FOR USE)   (TO BE PREPARED FOR USE)
(STRENGTH TO BE PREPARED)   (TOTAL TO BE PREPARED)

$$\text{dosage} : \text{amount} = \text{dosage} : \text{amount}$$
$$30 \text{ g} : 100 \text{ mL} = x \text{ g} : 2000 \text{ mL}$$
$$100x = 60,000$$
$$x = {}^{60,000}\!/_{100}$$
$$x = 600 \text{ g}$$

Step 2. Amount of solution needed

KNOWN AMOUNTS   **UNKNOWN AMOUNTS**
(AVAILABLE FOR USE)   (NEEDED TO BE USED)
(STRENGTH AVAILABLE)   (TOTAL TO BE PREPARED)

$$\text{dosage} : \text{amount} = \text{dosage} : \text{amount}$$
$$70 \text{ g} : 100 \text{ mL} = 600 \text{ g} : x \text{ mL}$$
$$70x = 60,000$$
$$x = {}^{60,000}\!/_{70}$$
$$x = 857\tfrac{1}{7} \text{ mL}$$

Answer: Use 857⅐ mL 70% alcohol and 1142⁶⁄₇ mL tap water to make a total volume of 2 qt of 30% alcohol for a cooling sponge immediately. (These amounts do not have to be measured this accurately, of course.)

Practice Problems

Answers can be found in Appendix C, p. 250.

Problem	Answer
1. ORDERED: NS enema stat (assume that one needs 1 qt of this solution) AVAILABLE: Sodium chloride crystals	
2. ORDERED: Irrigate both eyes with 3% sodium bicarbonate solution stat (one wants to prepare 2 qt of solution) AVAILABLE: Sodium bicarbonate powder	
3. ORDERED: Warm saturated boric acid solution compresses to lesions on right leg for 20 min qid (one needs 1 qt solution each treatment) AVAILABLE: Boric acid crystals and 1000 mL bottles of sterile water	

Problem	**Answer**

4. ORDERED: Rinse mouth with 2%
    sodium perborate qid (prepare
    100 mL each time)
   AVAILABLE: Sodium perborate
    powder

5. ORDERED: Sponge with 25%
    alcohol stat (one needs 2 qt of
    this solution)
   AVAILABLE: 1 pint bottles of
    70% isopropyl alcohol

6. ORDERED: 4 oz 2.5% dextrose
    solution PO q3h
   AVAILABLE: 50 mL ampules of
    50% dextrose and 500 mL and
    1000 mL bottles of 5% and
    10% dextrose

Problem	**Answer**

7. ORDERED: Hydrogen peroxide (3%) diluted 1:3 as mouthwash qid (one needs 1 oz each time)
   AVAILABLE: Hydrogen peroxide (3%) in 1 pt bottles

8. ORDERED: 1:3 alcohol sponge prn (one decides to use 1 pt of alcohol)
   AVAILABLE: 1 pt bottles of 70% isopropyl alcohol

9. ORDERED: Soak both feet in Dakin's solution (0.5%) for 15 min tid (one needs 2 qt for each treatment)
   AVAILABLE: Sodium hypochlorite solution 5% (Dakin's solution)

Problem	Answer

10. ORDERED: Irrigate left eye with
2% boric acid solution
(assume one wants to prepare
500 mL sterile solution)
AVAILABLE: Sterile 5% boric
acid solution

PART 12 • Other Nonparenteral Drugs

Suppositories are another common vehicle for administering medications. Suppositories can be administered via the rectum, vagina, or urethra. They are melted by the body temperature and absorption occurs locally. They are usually ordered in the doses that are available, and therefore no calculations are necessary. If they are to be halved, they should be cut lengthwise and not across.

Topical ointments also rely on local absorption. No calculations are necessary for this type of medication. However, specific directions should be read thoroughly and followed carefully.

Inhalation solutions require no calculations of specific dosages but three areas need careful attention by the health-care professional:

- Amount to be used
- Dilution specifications
- The method of administration by:
  ○ hand nebulizer, or,
  ○ oxygen or compressed air aerosolization, or,
  ○ intermittent positive pressure breathing (IPPB).

The drugs in this category are usually drugs that produce bronchodilatation and reduce bronchospasm. Figure 3–62 *A, B,* and *C* are examples of this type of medication.

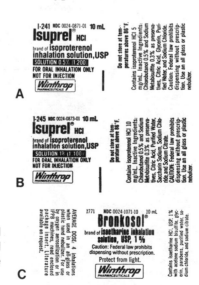

FIGURE 3–62 • Three inhalation solutions. **(A)** Isoproterenol (Courtesy of Winthrop Pharmaceuticals). **(B)** Isoproterenol (Courtesy of Winthrop Pharmaceuticals). **(C)** Isoetharine (Courtesy of Winthrop Pharmaceuticals).

CHAPTER 4

Parenteral Drugs

OBJECTIVES

At the end of this chapter, the student should be able to calculate accurately:
- The dosages of intradermal (ID), subcutaneous (SC or SQ), or intramuscular (IM):
  - drugs in solution
  - drugs requiring reconstitution
  - insulin
- The rate of flow and/or the amount of intravenous (IV) fluids and/or medications using:
  - primary sets
  - secondary sets
  - add-a-line sets
  - heparin locks
  - automatic controllers
  - volume delivery pumps
  - syringe infusers
- Fluid needs
- Calories in IV fluids

PART 13 • Drugs in Solution

Problems involving the parenteral administration of drugs are solved in exactly the same way as the oral solutions problems in Chapter 3. However, all answers are in minims (m) and/or milliliters (mL) because this is how syringes are calibrated. Drug strengths may be shown in any of the following ways:

gr/mL
mg/mL
g/mL
mEq/mL
U/mL

mcg/mL

percent (e.g., 1% or 1 g/100 mL)

ratio (e.g., 1:1000 or 1 g/1000 mL or 1 mg/1 mL)

The more common syringes that are available for parenteral dosages are illustrated in Figure 4–1.

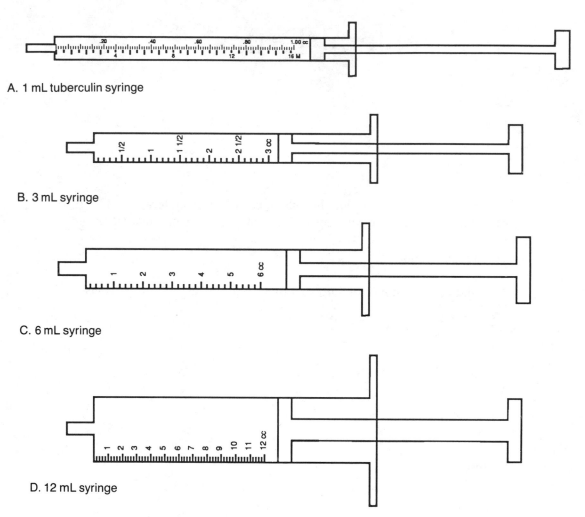

A. 1 mL tuberculin syringe

B. 3 mL syringe

C. 6 mL syringe

D. 12 mL syringe

FIGURE 4–1 • Syringes.

Example Problems

Problem 1: ORDERED: Tigan 150 mg IM qid

AVAILABLE: Trimethobenzamide hydrochloride (Tigan) 20 mL vial containing 200 mg/2 mL

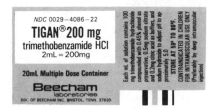

FIGURE 4–2 • Trimethobenzamide hydrochloride (Courtesy of Beecham Laboratories).

Solution: FORMULA B

KNOWN AMOUNTS   UNKNOWN AMOUNTS
(AVAILABLE FOR USE)   (ORDERED) (NEEDED)
$$\text{dosage:amount} = \text{dosage:amount}$$
$$200 \text{ mg:}2 \text{ mL} = 150 \text{ mg:}x \text{ mL}$$
$$200x = 300$$
$$x = {}^{300}\!/_{200}$$
$$x = 1.5 \text{ mL}$$

Answer: Administer 1.5 mL trimethobenzamide hydrochloride intramuscularly 4 times a day.

Problem 2: ORDERED: Demerol 20 mg IM q4h prn for pain
AVAILABLE: Meperidine hydrochloride (Demerol) 0.5 mL (25 mg) ampules

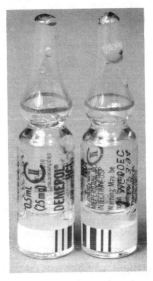

FIGURE 4–3 • Meperidine hydrochloride (From Winthrop Pharmaceuticals with permission).

Solution: FORMULA B

$$25 \text{ mg:}0.5 \text{ mL} = 20 \text{ mg:}x \text{ mL}$$
$$25x = 10$$
$$x = {}^{10}\!/_{25}$$
$$x = 0.4 \text{ mL}$$

Answer: Administer 0.4 mL meperidine hydrochloride intramuscularly every 4 hours when required for pain.

Problem 3: ORDERED: Neo-Synephrine 5 mg IM stat
AVAILABLE: Phenylephrine hydrochloride (Neo-Synephrine) 1% in 1 mL ampules

Neo-Synephrine® hydrochloride
brand of
phenylephrine hydrochloride injection, USP

1% STERILE AQUEOUS INJECTION

Each 1 mL contains
10 mg NEO-SYNEPHRINE hydrochloride, brand of phenylephrine hydrochloride, 3.5 mg sodium chloride, 4 mg sodium citrate, 1 mg citric acid monohydrate, and not more than 2 mg sodium metabisulfite as preservative.

FIGURE 4–4 • Phenylephrine hydrochloride (Courtesy of Winthrop Pharmaceuticals).

Solution:

$$1 \text{ g} : 100 \text{ mL, or}$$
$$1000 \text{ mg} : 100 \text{ mL, or}$$
$$1 \text{ mg} : 0.1 \text{ mL; so}$$
$$1 \text{ mg} : 0.1 \text{ mL} = 5 \text{ mg} : x \text{ mL}$$
$$1x = 0.1 \times 5$$
$$x = 0.5 \text{ mL}$$

Answer: Administer 0.5 mL phenylephrine hydrochloride 1% intramuscularly immediately.

Problem 4: ORDERED: Decadron 3 mg IM q6h

AVAILABLE: Dexamethasone sodium phosphate (Decadron) 4 mg/mL in a 1 mL vial

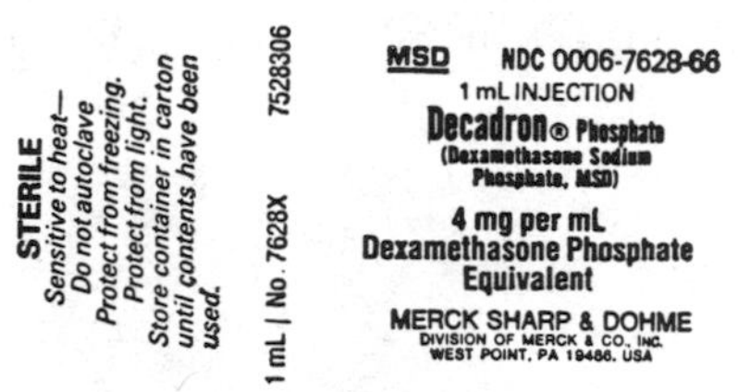

FIGURE 4–5 • Dexamethasone sodium phosphate (Courtesy of Merck Sharp & Dohme).

Solution:

$$4 \text{ mg} : 16 \text{ m } (1 \text{ mL}) = 3 \text{ mg} : x \text{ m}$$
$$4x = 48$$
$$x = {}^{48}\!/_4$$
$$x = 12 \text{ m}$$

Answer: Administer 12 m dexamethasone sodium phosphate intramuscularly every 6 hours.

Sixteen minims was used as the equivalent of 1 mL. Whenever drugs are given with a hypodermic or tuberculin syringe, use 16 m = 1 mL rather than 15 m = 1 mL when calculating the amount to be given. This gives a more accurate answer because these syringes are calibrated either with 16 m per mL or 16 plus m per mL, not with 15 m per mL. Hypodermic syringes are calibrated in tenths of a milliliter also. To give 1.25 mL, fill the syringe to the point halfway between 1.2 mL and 1.3 mL. To give 1.33 mL, fill the syringe to the point as nearly one third of the way between 1.3 and 1.4 mL as possible. Tuberculin syringes are calibrated in hundredths of a milliliter as well as in minims. When measuring small amounts (less than 1 mL) of parenteral solutions—for example, 2 m or 0.125 mL—use of a tuberculin syringe is desirable.

Problem 5: ORDERED: Heparin 8000 U SC q8h

AVAILABLE: Heparin sodium 10,000 U/mL in 1 mL vial

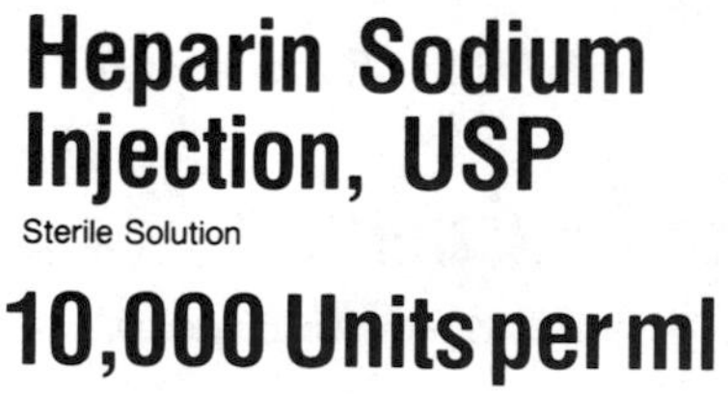

Heparin Sodium Injection, USP

Sterile Solution

10,000 Units per ml

FIGURE 4–6 • Heparin sodium (Courtesy of The Upjohn Company).

Solution:

$$10,000 \text{ U} : 1 \text{ mL} = 8000 \text{ U} : x \text{ mL}$$
$$10,000x = 8000$$
$$x = {}^{8000}\!/_{10,000}$$
$$x = 0.8 \text{ mL}$$

Answer: Administer 0.8 mL heparin sodium subcutaneously every 8 hours.

Problem 6: ORDERED: Zantac 40 mg IM q6h

AVAILABLE: Ranitidine hydrochloride (Zantac) 25 mg/mL in a 2 mL vial

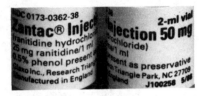

FIGURE 4–7 • Ranitidine hydrochloride (From Glaxo, Inc., with permission).

Solution:

$$25 \text{ mg} : 1 \text{ mL} = 40 \text{ mg} : x \text{ mL}$$
$$25x = 40$$
$$x = {}^{40}\!/_{25}$$
$$x = 1.6 \text{ mL}$$

Answer: Administer 1.6 mL of ranitidine hydrochloride intramuscularly every 6 hours.

Practice Problems:

Answers can be found in Appendix C, pp. 251–252.

Problem	Answer

1. ORDERED: Heparin 100 mg SC q8h

   AVAILABLE: A 4 mL vial of heparin sodium injection 10,000 U/mL (1 mg = 100 U)

NDC 0009-0317-02
One **4 ml** Vial

Heparin Sodium Injection, USP
Sterile Solution
10,000 Units per ml
from beef lung

For subcutaneous or intravenous use

Caution: Federal law prohibits dispensing without prescription.

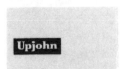

FIGURE 4–8 • Heparin sodium (Courtesy of The Upjohn Company).

2. ORDERED: Lanoxin 200 mcg IM at 0900 h

Problem   **Answer**

AVAILABLE: 2 mL ampules of
digoxin (Lanoxin) containing
500 mcg (0.5 mg)

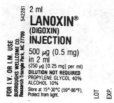

FIGURE 4–9 • Digoxin (Courtesy of Burroughs Wellcome Co.).

3. ORDERED: Cleocin 200 mg IM
   stat
   AVAILABLE: 4 mL vials of
   clindamycin phosphate
   (Cleocin) containing 600
   mg/4 mL

NDC 0009-0775-20   25—4 ml Vials (single dose containers)
6505-01-177-1982

Cleocin Phosphate® 600 mg
Sterile Solution
clindamycin phosphate injection, USP

Equivalent to **600 mg** clindamycin
For intramuscular or intravenous use
Caution: Federal law prohibits dispensing without prescription.

Upjohn

FIGURE   4–10 • Clindamycin   phosphate
(Courtesy of The Upjohn Company).

4. ORDERED: AquaMephyton 20 mg
   IM stat
   AVAILABLE: 1 mL ampules of
   phytonadione solution
   (AquaMephyton) 10 mg/mL

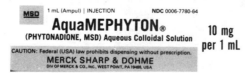

FIGURE 4–11 • Phytonadione (Courtesy of
Merck Sharp & Dohme).

Problem   **Answer**

5. ORDERED: Ranitidine
       hydrochloride 50 mg IM q8h
    AVAILABLE: Ranitidine
       hydrochloride (Zantac)
       25 mg/mL in 2 mL vial

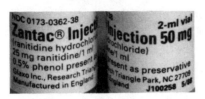

FIGURE 4–12 • Ranitidine hydrochloride
(From Glaxo, Inc., with permission).

6. ORDERED: Decadron 0.5 mg IM
       bid
    AVAILABLE: 1 mL vial
       containing 4 mg/mL of
       dexamethasone sodium
       phosphate (Decadron)

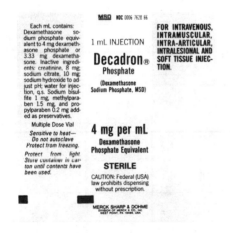

FIGURE 4–13 • Dexamethasone sodium
phosphate (Courtesy of Merck Sharp &
Dohme).

7. ORDERED: Morphine ¹⁄₁₀ gr SC
       q4h prn pain
    AVAILABLE: 1 mL ampules
       containing morphine sulfate
       8 mg (⅛ gr)/1 mL

Problem	Answer

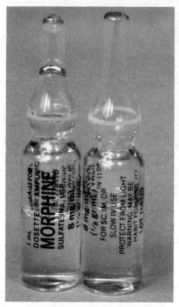

FIGURE 4–14 • Morphine sulfate (Courtesy of Elkins-Sinn, Inc.).

8. ORDERED: Robinul 0.1 mg IM
      qid
   AVAILABLE: 5 mL vial
      glycopyrrolate (Robinul)
      containing 0.2 mg/mL

5 mL Multiple Dose Vial   NDC 0031-7890-93
Robinul® Injectable
(Glycopyrrolate Injection, USP)
0.2 mg/mL
Water for Injection, USP q.s./Benzyl
Alcohol, NF (preservative) 0.9%.
[NOT FOR USE IN NEWBORNS]
pH adjusted, when necessary, with hydro-
chloric acid and/or sodium hydroxide.

CAUTION: Federal law prohibits dispens-
ing without prescription.
For I.M. or I.V. administration.
For dosage and other directions for use,
consult accompanying product literature.
Store at Controlled Room Temperature.
Between 15°C and 30°C (59°F and 86°F).
MANUFACTURED FOR   PHARMACEUTICAL DIVISION
A.H. ROBINS COMPANY, RICHMOND, VA. 23220
by ELKINS-SINN, INC., CHERRY HILL, N.J. 08003
a subsidiary of A.H. Robins   10.87

FIGURE 4–15 • Glycopyrrolate (Courtesy of A.H. Robins Company).

9. ORDERED: Neo-Synephrine 2 mg
      SC stat
   AVAILABLE: 1 mL ampule
      phenylephrine hydrochloride
      (Neo-Synephrine) 1%
      (10 mg/mL)

25 ampuls   1 mL (10 mg)

Neo-Synephrine® hydrochloride
brand of
phenylephrine hydrochloride injection, USP

1% STERILE AQUEOUS INJECTION

FIGURE 4–16 • Phenylephrine hydrochloride (Courtesy of Winthrop Pharmaceuticals).

Problem	**Answer**

10. ORDERED: Tigan 200 mg IM stat,
    then 100 mg IM q6h prn
    nausea
    AVAILABLE: 20 mL vial
    trimethobenzamide
    hydrochloride (Tigan)
    200 mg/2 mL

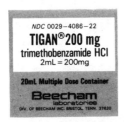

NDC 0029-4086-22
TIGAN®200 mg
trimethobenzamide HCl
2mL = 200mg

20mL Multiple Dose Container

Beecham
laboratories
DIV. OF BEECHAM INC. BRISTOL. TENN. 37620

FIGURE 4–17 • Trimethobenzamide hydrochloride (Courtesy of Beecham Laboratories).

11. ORDERED: Lasix 15 mg IM at
    0800 and 1400 h today
    AVAILABLE: Furosemide (Lasix)
    2 mL vial containing 20 mg

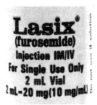

Lasix®
(furosemide)
Injection IM/IV
For Single Use Only
2 mL Vial
2 mL-20 mg(10 mg/mL)

FIGURE 4–18 • Furosemide (Courtesy of
Hoechst-Roussel Pharmaceuticals, Inc.).

12. ORDERED: Robinul 0.3 mg IM
    preoperatively at 1000 h
    AVAILABLE: 2 mL ampule
    glycopyrrolate (Robinul)
    0.2 mg/mL

NDC 0031-7890-95
Twenty-Five **2 ml** Single Dose Vials
Robinul®Injectable
(Glycopyrrolate Injection, USP)
0.4 mg/2 ml
(0.2 mg/ml)
Water for Injection, USP q.s./Benzyl
Alcohol, NF (preservative) 0.9%.
pH adjusted, when necessary, with hydro-
chloric acid and/or sodium hydroxide.

NOT FOR USE IN NEWBORNS
For I.M. or I.V. administration.

For dosage and other directions for
use, consult accompanying product
literature.
Store at Controlled Room Temperature, Between 15°C and 30°C (59°F
and 86°F).
CAUTION: Federal law prohibits dispensing without prescription.
MANUFACTURED FOR PHARMACEUTICAL DIVISION
A. H. ROBINS COMPANY, RICHMOND, VA. 23220
by ELKINS · SINN, INC., CHERRY HILL, N.J. 08003
a subsidiary of A.H. Robins   10.87

A·H·ROBINS

FIGURE 4–19 • Glycopyrrolate (Courtesy of
A.H. Robins).

Problem	**Answer**

13. ORDERED: Zantac 0.05 g IM q8h
    AVAILABLE: Ranitidine
    hydrochloride (Zantac)
    25 mg/mL in 40 mL
    bulk package

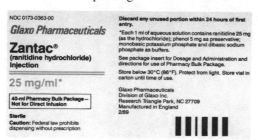

FIGURE 4–20 • Ranitidine hydrochloride (Courtesy of Glaxo, Inc).

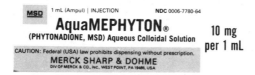

14. ORDERED: AquaMephyton
    0.005 g IM stat
    AVAILABLE: Phytonadione
    solution (AquaMephyton)
    10 mg/mL in 1 mL ampules

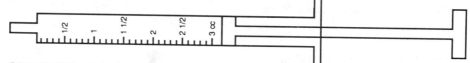

FIGURE 4–21 • Phytonadione (Courtesy of Merck Sharp & Dohme).

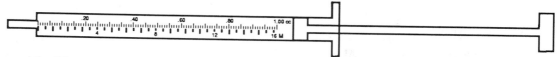

15. ORDERED: Lanoxin 100 mcg IM
    daily
    AVAILABLE: Digoxin (Lanoxin)
    0.5 mg/2 mL ampule

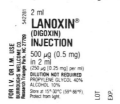

FIGURE 4–22 • Digoxin (Courtesy of Burroughs Wellcome Co.).

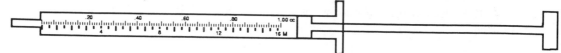

Problem	Answer

16. ORDERED: Tigan 0.1 g IM q4h
    AVAILABLE: Trimethobenzamide
    hydrochloride (Tigan)
    200 mg/2 mL in a 20 mL vial

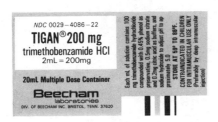

FIGURE 4–23 • Trimethobenzamide hydrochloride (Courtesy of Beecham Laboratories).

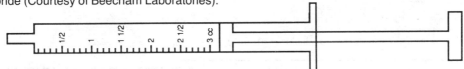

17. ORDERED: Vistaril 0.1 g IM stat
    and q6h
    AVAILABLE: Hydroxyzine
    hydrochloride (Vistaril)
    50 mg/mL in a 1 mL vial

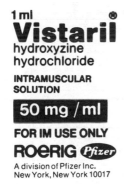

FIGURE 4–24 • Hydroxyzine hydrochloride
(Courtesy of Roerig).

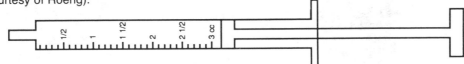

18. ORDERED: Morphine 1/16 gr SC
    q2–3h prn pain
    AVAILABLE: Morphine sulfate
    1/8 gr/mL in 1 mL ampule

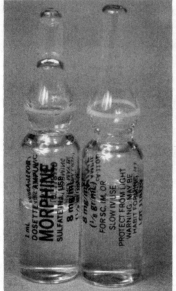

FIGURE 4–25 • Morphine sulfate (Courtesy of Elkins-Sinn, Inc.).

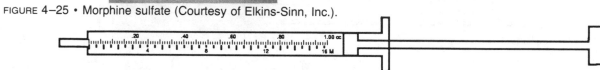

19. ORDERED: Robinul 0.3 mg IM preoperatively at 0600 h
    AVAILABLE: Glycopyrrolate (Robinul) in 2 mL vial with 0.2 mg/mL

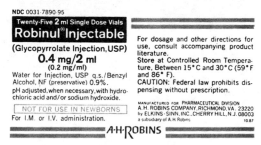

FIGURE 4–26 • Glycopyrrolate (Courtesy of A.H. Robins).

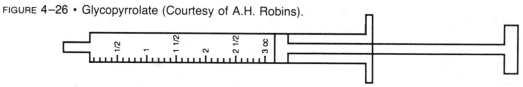

20. ORDERED: Lasix 20 mg IM at 0600 and 1400 h today only
    AVAILABLE: Furosemide (Lasix) 2 mL vial containing 20 mg

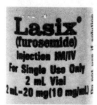

FIGURE 4–27 • Furosemide (Courtesy of Hoechst-Roussel Pharmaceuticals, Inc.).

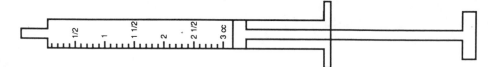

PART 14 • Drugs Requiring Reconstitution

Some penicillins, antibiotics, and other drugs to be given parenterally are stored in crystal or powder form in sterile vials or ampules. Before these drugs are administered, they must be dissolved in a desirable diluent or solvent, usually sterile isotonic saline or sterile distilled water labeled "for injection." A sterile syringe is used to withdraw the diluent from one sterile vial and to add it to the vial or ampule containing the drug in its dry form. After the drug has been dissolved in this diluent, the correct volume dose can be administered to the patient.

Please note: Multidose vials of sterile isotonic saline or sterile water for injection contain a bacteriostatic preservative that has been discovered to cause seizures in infants up to 1 month of age or more when such diluents are used to reconstitute drugs for intramuscular (IM) or intravenous (IV) use. Diluents that do not contain a preservative are available in single-dose vials and should be used when reconstituting drugs for use in nurseries and pediatric care units.

If the entire amount of drug in the vial is to be given at one time, simply add enough diluent to dissolve the drug, usually at least 1 to 2 mL, and give the entire amount. The amount needed to dissolve the drug varies with the type and amount of drug in the vial or ampule. Directions for dissolving drugs for parenteral administration usually can be found on the vial, on the box containing the vial, or on a pamphlet in the accompanying box. In some manner, these directions usually indicate the amount of volume that the drug itself occupies *after* it is in solution. For example, directions may say that adding 1.2 mL of sterile distilled water yields 2 mL of reconstituted solution. In other words, although the drug itself occupies considerably less space when in solution than when in dry form, this particular drug still displaces (occupies) 0.8 mL in volume measurement. In order to get 5 mL total volume of solution in this particular vial, one would add 4.2 mL of diluent, the drug occupies 0.8 mL so the resulting total volume would be 5 mL. If one added 5 mL diluent, there would be 5.8 mL in the vial.

Figures 4–28 *A* and *B* show that powders or crystals occupy a greater volume when in dry form than after they have been dissolved in a diluent.

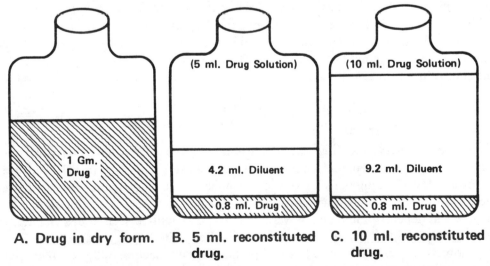

**A. Drug in dry form.   B. 5 ml. reconstituted   C. 10 ml. reconstituted
drug.   drug.**

FIGURE 4–28 • Displacement of 1 gram of drug. *(A)* Drug in dry form. *(B)* 5 mL of reconstituted drug. *(C)* 10 mL of reconstituted drug.

Figures 4–28 *B* and *C* show that when enough diluent to dissolve the drug has been added, the drug will occupy the same volume of space no matter how much more diluent is added. The drug will be dispersed throughout the total amount of solution.

In Figure 4–28 *B*, each milliliter of reconstituted drug solution contains one fifth of the 1 g of drug, or 200 mg. In Figure 4–28 *C*, each milliliter of reconstituted drug solution contains one tenth of the 1 g of drug, or 100 mg.

Figure 4–29 *A* shows one way that directions for reconstitution may be given. Adding 18.2 mL of diluent yields a solution of penicillin G sodium containing 250,000 U per mL and a total of 20 mL containing the total 5,000,000 U of the drug.

$$250,000 \text{ U}:1 \text{ mL} = 5,000,000 \text{ U}:x \text{ mL}$$
$$250,000x = 5,000,000$$
$$x = {}^{5,000,000}\!/_{250,000}$$
$$x = 20 \text{ mL}$$

The drug, therefore, occupies 1.8 mL of the 20 mL volume. If 3.2 mL of diluent were added, each milliliter of the prepared penicillin G solution would contain 1,000,000 U per mL. There would be 5 mL total solution, 1.8 mL of which would be the drug.

$$1,000,000 \text{ U}:1 \text{ mL} = 5,000,000 \text{ U}:x \text{ mL}$$
$$1,000,000x = 5,000,000$$
$$x = {}^{5,000,000}\!/_{1,000,000}$$
$$x = 5 \text{ mL}$$

Directions in Figure 4–29 *B* indicate that adding 1 mL of diluent will result in a solution of ampicillin containing 250 mg per mL. In such instances, the total amount of prepared solution will be slightly more than 1 mL. Therefore, there must be a little more than 250 mg of ampicillin in the vial.

$$250 \text{ mg}:1 \text{ mL} = x \text{ mg}:1^{+} \text{ mL}$$
$$x = 250^{+} \text{ mg}$$

Figure 4–29 *C* shows one of many variations of ready-to-mix vials in which the diluent is provided in the vial but separate from the drug in dry powder or crystal form. These vials provide a mechanism for releasing the diluent from the upper part of the vial into the lower part of the vial containing the drug in powder form. In this instance, addition of the diluent into the vial will yield approximately 3.0 mL of prepared cefazolin solution containing 330 mg per mL. Therefore, the vial contains approximately 1 g of cefazolin.

$$330 \text{ mg}:1 \text{ mL} = x \text{ mg}:3 \text{ mL}$$
$$x = 990 \text{ mg or 1 g}$$

Currently, very few drugs are given intramuscularly. Whenever possible, most drugs to be given parenterally are given intravenously. This is primarily because a therapeutic level of drug in the bloodstream can be attained and maintained more effectively via the intravenous route. Absorption of drugs from the muscle is quite unpredictable and dependent upon many variables. Also, as will be seen in this chapter, the amount that would be given intramuscularly is often quite large.

However, it should be noted that all problems in this section of this chapter are the same as the first step in the administration of drugs intravenously. That is, first, recon-

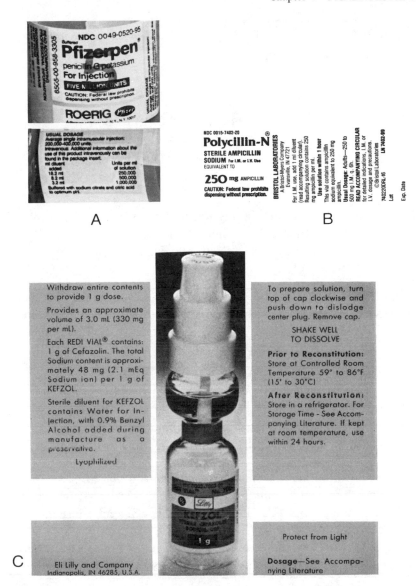

FIGURE 4–29 • Drugs requiring reconstitution. **(A)** Penicillin G potassium (From Roerig with permission). **(B)** Ampicillin sodium (Courtesy of Bristol Laboratories). **(C)** Cefazolin sodium (Courtesy of Eli Lilly and Company).

stitute the drug if necessary and, second, calculate the correct amount of reconstituted solution to use in order to give the ordered dosage of the drug.

All directions for the reconstitution of drugs given previously and hereafter are those actually found in the literature included in the packages of these drugs which are in current use. As will be seen, one must conclude that there apparently are occasional inconsistencies in the directions, or that the amount of the drug in the vial has been adjusted to make the directions accurate. Practicing pharmacists recommend following the directions on the literature in spite of the possible inconsistencies. Two of these possible inconsistencies follow. The calculations of drug displacements are ours. Apparent inconsistencies in drug displacement will be disregarded after these examples.

Example 1: DIRECTIONS: To get a concentration of approximately 500 mg/mL:

Add 1.5 mL diluent to 1 g vial
Add 5.7 mL diluent to 4 g vial
Add 8.6 mL diluent to 6 g vial

Solution:

$$\text{PREPARED} \quad \text{ORDERED}$$
$$500 \text{ mg} : 1 \text{ mL} = 1000 \text{ mg (1 g)} : x \text{ mL}$$
$$500x = 1000$$
$$x = {}^{1000}/_{500}$$
$$x = 2 \text{ mL}$$

Displacement: If there are 500 mg/mL in the 1 g vial after 1.5 mL of diluent has been added, there should be 2 mL of reconstituted solution. If so, the calculated drug displacement would be 0.5 mL for 1 g of dry drug.

DILUENT	VIAL	STRENGTH	CALCULATED VOLUME	CALCULATED DISPLACEMENT
1.5 mL	1 g	500 mg/mL	2 mL	0.5 mL
5.7 mL	4 g	500 mg/mL	8 mL	2.3 mL
8.6 mL	6 g	500 mg/mL	12 mL	3.4 mL

If there are 500 mg per mL in the 4 g vial after 5.7 mL of diluent were added, there should be 8 mL total volume of reconstituted solution. If so, the calculated drug displacement would be 2.3 mL (8 mL − 5.7 mL = 2.3 mL) instead of 2 mL as one would expect since 4 × 0.5 mL = 2 mL.

Likewise, if there are 500 mg per mL in the 6 g vial after 8.6 mL were added, there should be 12 mL total volume of reconstituted solution. If so, the calculated drug displacement would be 3.4 mL (12 mL − 8.6 mL = 3.4 mL) instead of 3 mL as one would expect, since 6 × 0.5 mL = 3 mL.

One can only follow the directions for the most appropriate concentration and hope that the margin of error, if any, does not exceed 10 percent.

Example 2: DIRECTIONS: Reconstitute as follows:

DILUENT	VIAL	MG/ML	CALCULATED VOLUME	CALCULATED DISPLACEMENT
3 mL	1 g	300	3.3 mL	0.3 mL
5 mL	2 g	330	6.1 mL	1.1 mL

Note that the displacement by 2 g of the drug is more than twice the displacement by 1 g of the drug.

Sometimes the vial contains more than one ordered dose. Whenever only a portion of the reconstituted drug is used, the vial should be properly labeled and dated so that the remaining drug may be given later yet before the expiration time of the reconstituted drug. Because the ordered dosage is often available in 1 mL, it is a safety precaution to label vials with the dosage per milliliter; for example, ''200,000 U per mL'' or ''0.5 g per mL,'' even though the ordered dosage may be less or more than the amount of drug in 1 mL.

Most drugs should be refrigerated after reconstitution. Drug pamphlets tell how long the drug remains stable at room temperature or refrigerated. Therefore, place the date and time of reconstitution on the label along with the dosage as stated earlier. Many agencies require practitioners to put their names on the labels of drugs that they reconstitute.

All parenteral solutions problems can be solved with the proportion Formula B, starting with the amounts that are known to be available for, or which have been prepared for, use. It may be necessary to use Formula A first if the ordered and available dosages are not in the same unit of measurement.

Example Problems

Problem 1: ORDERED: Penicillin G 2,000,000 U IM q3h

AVAILABLE: Penicillin G potassium (Pfizerpen) vial containing 5,000,000 U in dry form

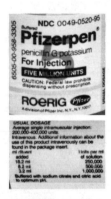

FIGURE 4–30 • Penicillin G potassium (From Roerig with permission).

DIRECTIONS: Reconstitute as follows:

DILUENT	U/ML
18.2 mL	250,000
8.2 mL	500,000
3.2 mL	1,000,000

Solution:

KNOWN AMOUNTS	UNKNOWN AMOUNTS
(PREPARE FOR USE)	(ORDERED) (NEEDED)

$$1,000,000 \text{ U}:1 \text{ mL} = 2,000,000 \text{ U}:x \text{ mL}$$
$$1,000,000x = 2,000,000$$
$$x = {}^{2,000,000}\!/_{1,000,000}$$
$$x = 2 \text{ mL}$$

Answer: Add 3.2 mL of diluent to the 5,000,000 U vial and give 2 mL intramuscularly every 3 hours. There will be two and one-half doses in this vial.

$$2,000,000 \text{ U}:1 \text{ dose} = 5,000,000 \text{ U}:x \text{ dose(s)}$$
$$2,000,000x = 5,000,000$$
$$x = {}^{5,000,000}\!/_{2,000,000}$$
$$x = 2\tfrac{1}{2} \text{ doses}$$

Problem 2: ORDERED: Penicillin G 300,000 U IM q2h
AVAILABLE: Same as Problem 1
DIRECTIONS: Same as Problem 1

Solution: Select one or more concentrations in the directions that are the closest to the ordered dosage; for example, 250,000 U/mL or 500,000 U/mL.

$$250,000 \text{ U} : 1 \text{ mL} = 300,000 \text{ U} : x \text{ mL}$$
$$250,000x = 300,000$$
$$x = {}^{300,000}/_{250,000}$$
$$x = 1.2 \text{ mL}$$
$$\text{or}$$
$$500,000 \text{ U} : 1 \text{ mL} = 300,000 \text{ U} : x \text{ mL}$$
$$500,000x = 300,000$$
$$x = {}^{300,000}/_{500,000}$$
$$x = 0.6 \text{ mL}$$

Answer: Two actions would be reasonable:

• Add 18.2 mL of diluent to this vial and give 1.2 mL intramuscularly every 2 hours.
• Add 8.2 mL of diluent and give 0.6 mL intramuscularly every 2 hours.

Problem 3: ORDERED: Penicillin G potassium 300,000 U IM q2h
AVAILABLE: Penicillin G potassium (Pfizerpen) vial containing 1,000,000 U in dry form

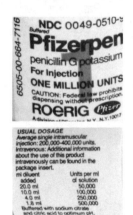

FIGURE 4–31 • Penicillin G potassium (From Roerig with permission).

DIRECTIONS: Reconstitute as follows:

DILUENT	U/mL
20.0 mL	50,000
10.0 mL	100,000
4.0 mL	250,000
1.8 mL	500,000

Solution:

$$250,000 \text{ U} : 1 \text{ mL} = 300,000 \text{ U} : x \text{ mL}$$
$$250,000x = 300,000$$
$$x = {}^{300,000}/_{250,000}$$
$$x = 1.2 \text{ mL}$$

or

$$500,000 \text{ U}:1 \text{ mL} = 300,000 \text{ U}:x \text{ mL}$$
$$500,000x = 300,000$$
$$x = {}^{300,000}\!/_{500,000}$$
$$x = 0.6 \text{ mL}$$

Answer: Two actions would be acceptable, although the second results in a smaller volume to be given to the patient:

- Add 4.0 mL of diluent to this vial and give 1.2 mL intramuscularly every 2 hours.

or

- Add 1.8 mL of diluent and give 0.6 mL intramuscularly every 2 hours.

In either instance, since there are 1,000,000 U in this vial and 300,000 U are ordered, there are three and one-third doses in this vial.

$$300,000 \text{ U}:1 \text{ dose} = 1,000,000 \text{ U}:x \text{ doses}$$
$$300,000x = 1,000,000$$
$$x = {}^{1,000,000}\!/_{300,000}$$
$$x = 3\frac{1}{3} \text{ doses}$$

Problem 4: ORDERED: Mefoxin 800 mg IM q4h

AVAILABLE: Cefoxitin sodium (Mefoxin) vials containing 1 g and 2 g of dry powder

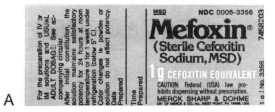 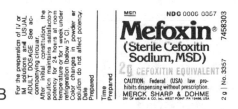

FIGURE 4–32 • Cefoxitin sodium. **(A)** 1g and **(B)** 2 g (Courtesy of Merck Sharp & Dohme).

DIRECTIONS: Reconstitute as follows:

STRENGTH	DILUENT	APPROXIMATE WITHDRAWAL	APPROXIMATE CONCENTRATION
1 g	2 mL	2.5 mL	400 mg/mL
2 g	4 mL	5.0 mL	400 mg/mL

Solution:

$$400 \text{ mg}:1 \text{ mL} = 800 \text{ mg}:x \text{ mL}$$
$$400x = 800$$
$$x = {}^{800}\!/_{400}$$
$$x = 2 \text{ mL}$$

Answer: Add 2 mL of diluent to the 1 g vial and give 2 mL intramuscularly every 4 hours, or add 4 mL to the 2 g vial and give 2 mL intramuscularly every 4 hours. There would be one and one-fourth doses in the 1 g vial and two and one-half doses in the 2 g vial.

Problem 5: ORDERED: Ticar 500 mg IM q6h

AVAILABLE: Ticarcillin disodium (Ticar) 6 g vial

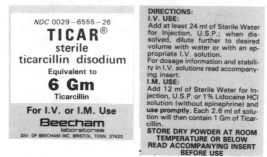

FIGURE 4–33 • Ticarcillin disodium (Courtesy of Beecham Laboratories).

DIRECTIONS: For IM use, add 12 mL diluent to the 6 g vial and each 2.6 mL of solution will contain 1 g of drug.

Solution:
$$2.6 \text{ mL}:1 \text{ g} = x \text{ mL}:0.5 \text{ g}$$
$$1x = 2.6 \times 0.5$$
$$x = 1.3 \text{ mL}$$

Answer: Add 12 mL of recommended diluent to the 6 g vial and give 1.3 mL intramuscularly every 6 hours.

Problem 6: ORDERED: Unasyn 1.5 g IM q6h

AVAILABLE: Ampicillin sodium 1 g and sulbactam sodium 0.5 g (Unasyn 1.5 g)

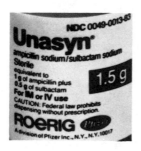

FIGURE 4–34 • Ampicillin sodium/subactam sodium (From Roerig with permission).

DIRECTIONS: Adding 3.2 mL of appropriate diluent to the 1.5 g vial yields 4 mL of reconstituted solution containing Unasyn 375 mg/mL.

Solution: Amount ordered equals the amount available.

Answer: Add 3.2 mL of diluent to the 1.5 g vial and give the entire resulting solution to give 1.5 g of Unasyn intramuscularly every 6 hours. Give within 1 hour.

Practice Problems

Answers can be found in Appendix C, pp. 252–254.

Problem	Answer
1. ORDERED: Mefoxin 2 g IM at 0630 h preoperatively AVAILABLE: Cefoxitin sodium (Mefoxin) 2 g vial	

Problem	**Answer**

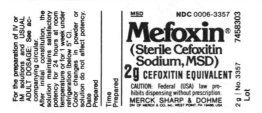

FIGURE 4–35 • Cefoxitin sodium (Courtesy of Merck Sharp & Dohme).

DIRECTIONS: For IM use, add
4 mL of diluent to the 2 g vial
to get 5 mL of drug solution
with 400 mg/mL.

2. ORDERED: Polycillin-N 500 mg
    IM q6h
   AVAILABLE: Ampicillin sodium
    (Polycillin-N) in dry form in
    1 g vial

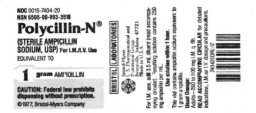

FIGURE 4–36 • Ampicillin sodium (Courtesy of Bristol Laboratories).

DIRECTIONS: For IM use, add
3.5 mL of diluent. Resulting
solution contains ampicillin
250 mg/mL.

3. ORDERED: Claforan 0.5 g IM q6h
   AVAILABLE: Cefotaxime sodium
    (Claforan) in dry form in a
    1 g vial

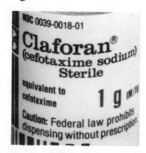

FIGURE 4–37 • Cefotaxime sodium (From Hoechst-Roussel Pharmaceuticals, Inc. with permission).

Problem   **Answer**

DIRECTIONS: Add 3 mL diluent
to a 1 g vial to get 3.4 mL of
reconstituted drug containing
approximately 300 mg/mL.

4. ORDERED: Claforan 0.75 g IM
    preoperatively in AM
    AVAILABLE: Same as in
    Problem 3
    DIRECTIONS: Same as in
    Problem 3

5. ORDERED: Prostaphlin 250 mg
    IM q4h
    AVAILABLE: Oxacillin sodium
    (Prostaphlin) in dry form in
    250 mg vial

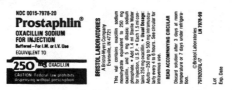

FIGURE 4–38 • Oxacillin sodium (Courtesy of
Bristol Laboratories).

DIRECTIONS: To obtain a
solution containing 250 mg of
drug in 1.5 mL of solution,
add 1.4 mL of diluent.

6. ORDERED: Kefzol 250 mg IM stat
    and q6h
    AVAILABLE: Cefazolin sodium
    (Kefzol) in dry form in 250
    mg vials

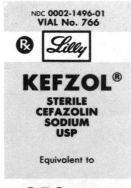

FIGURE 4–39 • Cefazolin sodium (Courtesy
of Eli Lilly and Company).

Problem	Answer

DIRECTIONS: Adding 2 mL
diluent yields approximately
2 mL (125 mg/mL).

7. ORDERED: Pfizerpen 500,000 U
   IM q4h
   AVAILABLE: Penicillin G
   potassium (Pfizerpen)
   1,000,000 U vial

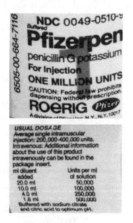

FIGURE 4–40 • Penicillin G potassium (From Roerig with permission).

DIRECTIONS: Reconstitute as
follows:

DILUENT	U/mL
20.0 mL	50,000
10.0 mL	100,000
4.0 mL	250,000
1.8 mL	500,000

8. ORDERED: Unasyn 1 g IM q4h
   AVAILABLE: Ampicillin sodium
   1 g and sulbactam sodium
   0.5 g (Unasyn 1.5 g) dry
   powder in 1.5 g vial

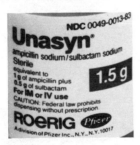

FIGURE 4–41 • Ampicillin sodium/sulbactam sodium (From Roerig with permission).

Problem	**Answer**

DIRECTIONS: For IM, adding
3.2 mL of diluent yields 4 mL
(375 mg/mL). Give within
1 h.

9. ORDERED: Pfizerpen 1,000,000 U
IM q6h
AVAILABLE: Penicillin G
potassium (Pfizerpen)
5,000,000 U

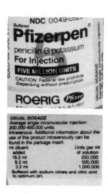

FIGURE 4–42 • Penicillin G potassium (From Roerig with permission).

DIRECTIONS: Reconstitute as
follows:

DILUENT	U/mL
18.2 mL	250,000
8.2 mL	500,000
3.2 mL	1,000,000

10. ORDERED: Staphcillin 1 g IM q4h
AVAILABLE: Methicillin sodium
(Staphcillin) in dry form in
6 g vial

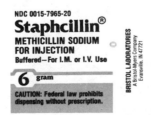

FIGURE 4–43 • Methicillin sodium (Courtesy of Bristol Laboratories).

Problem	**Answer**

DIRECTIONS: For IM use, add
8.6 mL of diluent and each
2 mL will contain 1 g
of Staphcillin.

11. ORDERED: Pipracil 2 g IM stat
AVAILABLE: Piperacillin sodium
(Pipracil) in dry form in
2 g vial

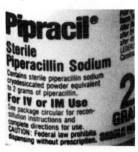

FIGURE 4–44 • Piperacillin sodium (From Lederle Laboratories with permission).

DIRECTIONS: Use no more than
2 g per injection site.
Reconstitute every gram with
a minimum of 2 mL of
diluent. Adding 4 mL of
diluent yields 1g/2.5 mL
of solution.

12. ORDERED: Kefzol 1 g IM q6h
AVAILABLE: Cefazolin sodium
(Kefzol) dry power in 1 g vial

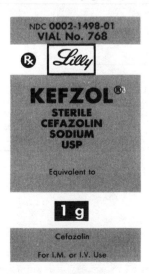

FIGURE 4–45 • Cefazolin sodium (Courtesy of Eli Lilly and Company).

Problem	**Answer**

DIRECTIONS: Add 2.5 mL of
sterile water to get
approximately 3 mL
(330 mg/mL).

Indicate the dosage of each drug on the syringe provided in the answer column.

13. ORDERED: Mefoxin 0.6 g IM qid
     AVAILABLE: Cefoxitin sodium
         (Mefoxin) 1 g and 2 g vials of
         dry powder

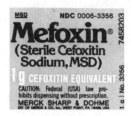
A

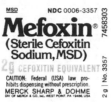
B

FIGURE 4–46 • Cefoxitin sodium. **(A)** 1 g and **(B)** 2 g (Courtesy of Merck Sharp & Dohme).

DIRECTIONS:

STRENGTH	DILUENT	APPROX-IMATE WITH-DRAWAL	APPROX-IMATE CONCEN-TRATION
1 g	2 mL	2.5 mL	400 mg/mL
2 g	4 mL	5.0 mL	400 mg/mL

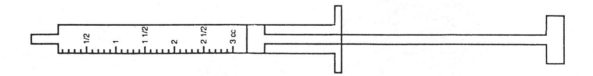

14. ORDERED: Ticar 800 mg IM q6h
     AVAILABLE: Ticarcillin disodium
         (Ticar) 6 g dry powder in
         a vial

Problem   **Answer**

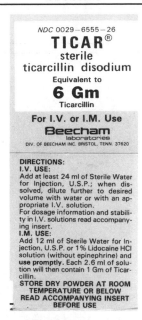

FIGURE 4–47 • Ticarcillin disodium (Courtesy of Beecham Laboratories).

DIRECTIONS: For IM use, add
12 mL diluent to a 6 g vial
and each 2.6 mL of solution
will contain 1 g of drug.

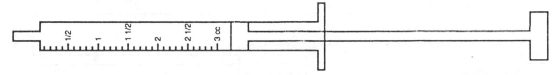

15. ORDERED: Polycillin-N 0.75 g
IM q6h
AVAILABLE: Ampicillin sodium
(Polycillin-N) in dry form in a
1 g vial

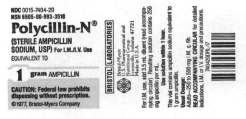

FIGURE 4–48 • Ampicillin sodium (Courtesy of Bristol Laboratories).

DIRECTIONS: For IM use, add
3.5 mL to 1 g vial. Resulting
solution contains 250 mg/mL.

Problem	Answer

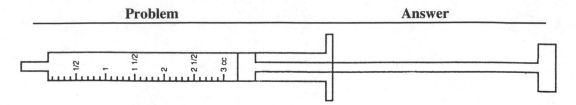

16. ORDERED: Claforan 800 mg
    IM q6h
    AVAILABLE: Cefotaxime sodium
    (Claforan) in dry form in a 1 g
    vial

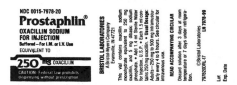

FIGURE 4–49 • Cefotaxime sodium (From Hoechst-Roussel Pharmaceuticals, Inc. with permission).

DIRECTIONS: Add 3 mL diluent
to a 1 g vial to get 3.4 mL of
reconstituted drug containing
approximately 300 mg/mL.

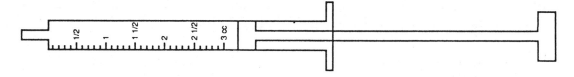

17. ORDERED: Prostaphlin 0.5 g
    IM q4h
    AVAILABLE: Oxacillin sodium
    (Prostaphlin) in dry form in a
    250 mg vial

FIGURE 4–50 • Oxacillin sodium (Courtesy of Bristol Laboratories).

DIRECTIONS: To obtain a
solution containing 250 mg of
drug in 1.5 mL of solution,

Problem	Answer

add 1.4 mL of diluent to the
250 mg vial.

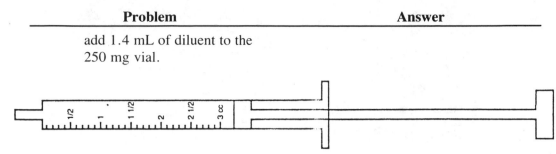

18. ORDERED: Kefzol 0.125 g
    IM q4h
    AVAILABLE: Cefazolin sodium
    (Kefzol) in dry form in
    250 mg vials

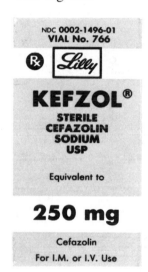

FIGURE 4–51 • Cefazolin sodium (Courtesy
of Eli Lilly and Company).

DIRECTIONS: Adding 1 mL of
    diluent yields approximately
    2 mL of solution.

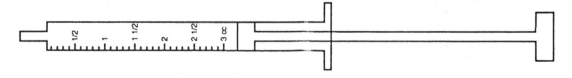

19. ORDERED: Pfizerpen 125,000 U
    IM q4h
    AVAILABLE: Penicillin G
    potassium (Pfizerpen)
    1,000,000 U in dry form in
    a vial

Problem   **Answer**

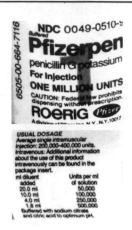

FIGURE 4–52 • Penicillin G potassium (From Roerig with permission).

DIRECTIONS: Reconstitute
    1,000,000 U vial as follows:

DILUENT	U/ML
20.0 mL	50,000
10.0 mL	100,000
4.0 mL	250,000
1.8 mL	500,000

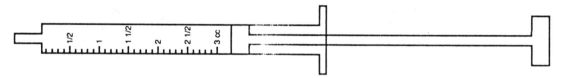

20. ORDERED: Staphcillin 600 mg
       IM q4h
    AVAILABLE: Methicillin sodium
       (Staphcillin) in dry form in
       6 g vial

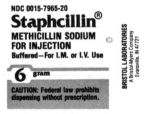

FIGURE 4–53 • Methicillin sodium (Courtesy of Bristol Laboratories).

DIRECTIONS: For IM use, add
       8.6 mL of diluent and each
       2 mL will contain 1 g
       of staphcillin.

Problem	Answer

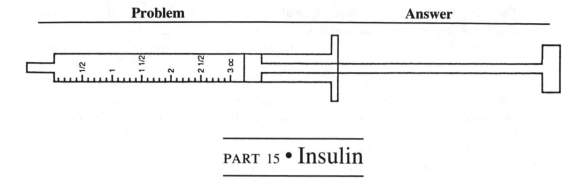

PART 15 • Insulin

This section, like the section on Preparing Solutions for Topical Use, is presented more for information than for the practice in calculations of insulin dosages. Primarily only 100 units per milliliter (U/mL) insulin is used in the United States.

The past 10 years have provided many improvements in insulin with respect to source, purity, concentrations, dosage requirements, and methods of administration.

One of the major advances was the synthesis of human insulin using bacteria genetically altered by recombinant DNA technology. It is a purer form of insulin and causes fewer side effects. In addition, it can be used by persons with sensitivities to the beef and pork insulins that have been available for many years.

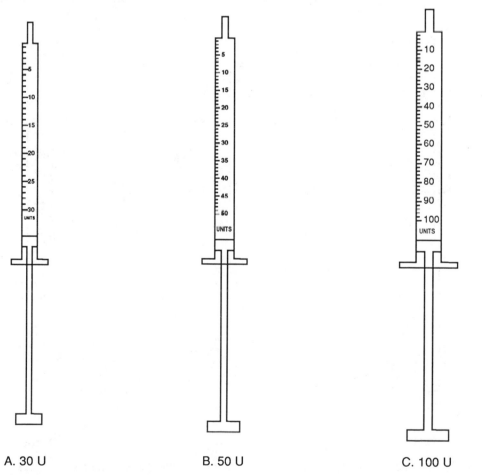

A. 30 U   B. 50 U   C. 100 U

FIGURE 4–54 • Insulin syringes. **(A)** 0.3 mL (30 U). **(B)** 0.5 mL (50 U). **(C)** 1.0 mL (100 U).

There are four main categories of insulin, which are based on rapidity of onset available from human, beef, and pork sources: rapid-acting (onset ½ to 4 hours), intermediate-acting (onset 1 to 4 hours), a premixture of rapid-acting and intermediate-acting (onset ½ to 4 hours), and long-acting (onset 4 to 6 hours). It is not within the scope of this book to discuss these in detail. The type of insulin and the dosage amounts of insulin needed by each individual patient are determined by the physician.

The most common method of administration of insulin is by the subcutaneous (SC) route, using the standard insulin syringes which are available in 30 U (0.3 mL), 50 U (0.5 mL), and 100 U per mL (1.0 mL) as shown in Figure 4–54. Unless otherwise noted, all insulin injections are to be given subcutaneously.

An aspect of insulin injection that needs careful attention is the depth of the tissue into which the needle is to be injected. The standard needle on an insulin syringe is ⅝ inch long. Since the desired site of injection is the subcutaneous tissue, the amount of fatty tissue through which the needle must pass in order to reach the subcutaneous tissue should be judged by the practitioner giving the injection. If more than ⅜ inch of fatty tissue is judged to be present, a longer needle should be used for the injection. If the insulin is injected into the fatty tissue, it will not be absorbed well since fatty tissue has fewer blood vessels for absorption.

If it is desired that the insulin should have a more rapid absorption, an intramuscu-

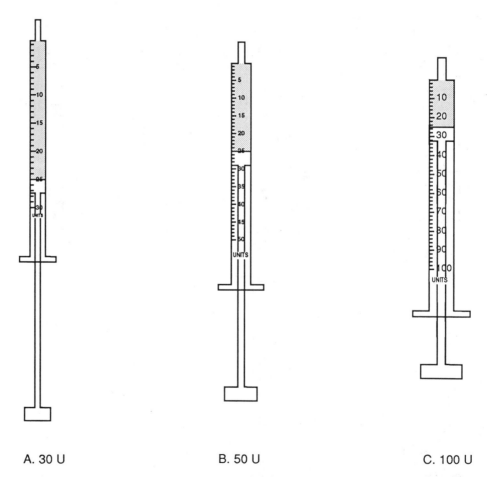

A. 30 U   B. 50 U   C. 100 U

FIGURE 4–55 • Insulin dose of 25 units. **(A)** In a 0.3 mL syringe. **(B)** In a 0.5 mL syringe. **(C)** In a 1.0 mL syringe.

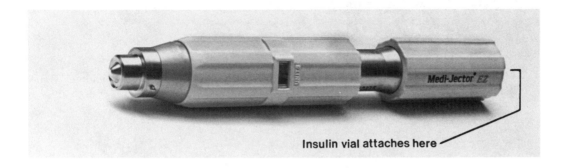

Insulin vial attaches here

FIGURE 4–56 • Derata Medi-Jector EZ syringe (Courtesy of Derata Corporation).

lar (IM) route may be ordered and a longer needle used for this injection to reach the muscular tissue, again being sure to consider the fatty tissue the needle must penetrate. Injection via this route is seen only occasionally.

Because insulin is available in 100 U per mL, the amount of insulin ordered is the same as the amount to be measured into a 30 U (0.3 mL), a 50 U (0.5 mL), or a 100 U (1.0 mL) insulin syringe. For example, if 25 U of insulin is ordered, the insulin would be drawn into the insulin syringe to the 25 U mark in each of the three syringe sizes, as illustrated in Figure 4–55.

To ensure the most accurate dose possible, a 0.3 mL syringe should be used for insulin dosages under 30 U; a 0.5 mL syringe for insulin dosages 30 to 50 U; and a 1.0 mL syringe for insulin dosages more than 50 U.

Two of the newer syringe-type methods of administering insulin are the Medi-Jector EZ (Fig. 4–56) manufactured by Derata Corporation and the NovolinPen (Fig. 4–58) manufactured by Squibb-Novo, Incorporated.

The Medi-Jector EZ syringe is pictured approximately one-half its actual size. The syringe may appear to be large and cumbersome, but it has several advantages over the conventional syringe. The insulin vial is attached directly to the syringe before each initial dose from that vial and remains there until the last dose from that vial is given. This cuts down on the number of chances for contamination and the number of times that errors in the dosage might be made. It also allows people with diminished vision to safely administer a preset dosage of insulin.

Perhaps one of the most important advantages of the Medi-Jector EZ is the way the medication is injected into the subcutaneous tissue when administered by this jet pressure-propelled syringe (Fig. 4–57). With this type of dispersion of medication into the subcutaneous tissue, the absorption should be faster and the local tissue trauma lessened.

The Squibb-Novo Novolin Pen insulin delivery device is a more conventional-sized device that comes with individual Dial-a-Dose PenFill cartridges to allow the administration of preset doses of insulin, and, therefore, has the same advantages as the

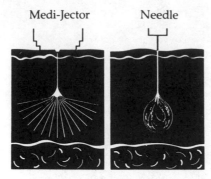

FIGURE 4–57 • Comparative dispersion patterns (Courtesy of Derata Corporation).

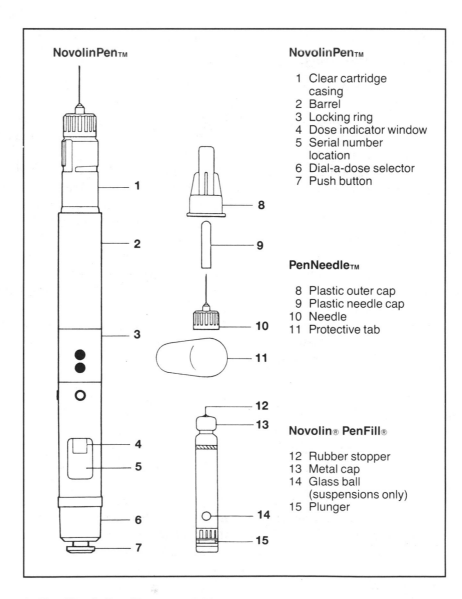

NovolinPen™

NovolinPen™

1 Clear cartridge casing
2 Barrel
3 Locking ring
4 Dose indicator window
5 Serial number location
6 Dial-a-dose selector
7 Push button

PenNeedle™

8 Plastic outer cap
9 Plastic needle cap
10 Needle
11 Protective tab

Novolin® PenFill®

12 Rubber stopper
13 Metal cap
14 Glass ball (suspensions only)
15 Plunger

FIGURE 4–58 • NovolinPen (Courtesy of Squibb-Nova, Inc.).

TABLE 4.1 • **Types of Insulin Available in 1990**			
Product	*Manufacturer*	*Form*	*Strength*
Rapid-Acting (Onset ½–4 Hours)			
Humulin Regular	Lilly	Human	U-100
Humulin BR (for external insulin pumps only)	Lilly	Human	U-100
Novolin R (Regular)	Squibb-Novo	Human	U-100
Velosulin Human (Regular)	Nordisk-USA	Human	U-100
Iletin II Regular	Lilly	Beef	U-100
Iletin II Regular	Lilly	Pork	U-100, U-500
Purified Pork R (Regular)	Squibb-Novo	Pork	U-100
Velosulin (Regular)	Nordisk-USA	Pork	U-100
Purified Pork S (Semilente)	Squibb-Novo	Pork	U-100
Iletin I Regular	Lilly	Beef/Pork	U-40, U-100
Regular	Squibb-Novo	Pork	U-100
Iletin I Semilente	Lilly	Beef/Pork	U-40, U-100
Semilente	Squibb-Novo	Beef	U-100
Novolin R Penfill (Regular)	Squibb-Novo	Human	U-100
Intermediate-Acting (Onset 1–4 Hours)			
Humulin L	Lilly	Human	U-100
Humulin NPH	Lilly	Human	U-100
Insulatard Human NPH	Nordisk-USA	Human	U-100
Novolin L (Lente)	Squibb-Novo	Human	U-100
Novolin N (NPH)	Squibb-Novo	Human	U-100
Novolin NPH Penfill (NPH)	Squibb-Novo	Human	U-100
Iletin II Lente	Lilly	Beef	U-100
Iletin II NPH	Lilly	Beef	U-100
Iletin II Lente	Lilly	Pork	U-100
Iletin II NPH	Lilly	Pork	U-100
Insulatard NPH	Nordisk-USA	Pork	U-100
Purified Pork Lente	Squibb-Novo	Pork	U-100
Purified Pork N (NPH)	Squibb-Novo	Pork	U-100
Lente	Squibb-Novo	Beef	U-100
Iletin I Lente	Lilly	Beef/Pork	U-40, U-100
Iletin I NPH	Lilly	Beef/Pork	U-40, U-100
NPH	Squibb-Novo	Beef	U-100
Long-Acting (Onset 4–6 Hours)			
Iletin II PZI	Lilly	Beef	U-100
Iletin II PZI	Lilly	Pork	U-100
Purified Beef U (Ultralente)	Squibb-Novo	Beef	U-100
Iletin I PZI	Lilly	Beef/Pork	U-40, U-100
Iletin I Ultralente	Lilly	Beef/Pork	U-40, U-100
Ultralente	Squibb-Novo	Beef	U-100
Humulin U (Ultralente)	Lilly	Human	U-100
Mixtures			
Mixtard (30% Regular, 70% NPH)	Nordisk-USA	Pork	U-100
Mixtard Human 70/30 (70% NPH Human, 30% Regular Human)	Nordisk-USA	Human	U-100
Novolin 70/30 (70% NPH, 30% Regular)	Squibb-Novo	Human	U-100
Novolin 70/30 Penfill	Squibb-Novo	Human	U-100
Humulin 70/30 (70% NPH, 30% Regular)	Lilly	Human	U-100

Reprinted with permission from Diabetes Forecast, October 1989. Copyright © 1989 American Diabetes Association, Inc.

Medi-Jector, decreasing the number of chances for contamination and dosage error. However, the pattern of dispersion of medication in the NovolinPen is the same as that of a conventional insulin syringe. It is primarily used for small doses of supplemental regular insulin during the day which can be administered in 2 U increments.

Different methods of administration of insulin are continuously being studied in an attempt to find the safest, most convenient, and efficient way to administer insulin. One method, an open-loop system, is the external insulin pump, which is worn externally and administers preset amounts of regular insulin into the subcutaneous tissue. Another method, a closed-loop system, is the internal insulin pump, which is implanted surgically and has a programmable system that controls the injection of insulin. The latter method is now being researched in human subjects.

There are many types of insulin available, as shown in Table 4–1. Insulin 100 U per mL is used in most instances, but 40 U per mL and 500 U per mL insulin types are available for use in special situations.

Because doses of insulin are very small and need to be measured exactly, *every effort possible should be made to obtain an appropriately calibrated insulin syringe.* Only in emergency or disaster situations when the needs of the patient outweigh the delay in obtaining an appropriately calibrated insulin syringe should any other type of syringe be used. Examples are given for calculation of insulin doses when insulin syringes are not available and standard tuberculin and 3 mL syringes are available for use.

Example Problems

Problem 1: ORDERED: Novolin R insulin 80 U deep SC stat
AVAILABLE: Regular human insulin (Novolin R) 100 U/mL and no insulin syringe

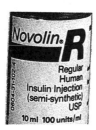

FIGURE 4–59 • Regular human insulin (Courtesy of Squibb-Nova, Inc.).

Solution: FORMULA B

$$
\begin{array}{cc}
\textbf{KNOWN AMOUNTS} & \textbf{UNKNOWN AMOUNTS} \\
\text{(AVAILABLE FOR USE)} & \text{(ORDERED) (NEEDED)} \\
\text{dosage : amount} & \text{dosage : amount}
\end{array}
$$

$$100 \text{ U} : 1 \text{ mL} = 80 \text{ U} : x \text{ mL}$$
$$100x = 80$$
$$x = {}^{80}\!/_{100}$$
$$x = 0.8 \text{ mL}$$

or

$$100 \text{ U} : 16 \text{ m} = 80 \text{ U} : x \text{ m}$$
$$100x = 16 \times 80$$
$$100x = 1280$$
$$x = {}^{1280}\!/_{100}$$
$$x = 12.8 \text{ m}$$

Answer: Use a tuberculin syringe and give 0.8 mL or 12.8 m regular human insulin immediately, deep subcutaneously. (These two measurements should be at the same point on the tuberculin syringe.)

Tuberculin syringes have a 1 mL volume. They have two scales: one is calibrated in hundredths of a milliliter (100 hundredths/mL) and the other in minims (16 m/mL). When small volumes of insulin are to be given, the correct dosage can be measured more accurately when using a tuberculin syringe rather than a 3 mL (standard volume) hypodermic syringe. The standard volume 3 mL hypodermic syringes would never be used to measure insulin unless there was an emergency that prohibited obtaining an insulin or a tuberculin syringe.

Sometimes two kinds of insulin are given at the same time, as in Problem 2.

Problem 2: ORDERED: Novolin R 16 U and Novolin N 30 U SC ac qAM
AVAILABLE: Regular human insulin (Novolin R) 100 U/mL and NPH human insulin isophane suspension (Novolin N) 100 U/mL and no insulin syringe

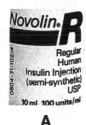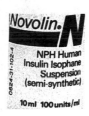

A   **B**

FIGURE 4–60 • **(A)** Regular human insulin and **(B)** NPH human insulin isophane suspension (Courtesy of Squibb-Nova, Inc.).

Solution:

$$100 \text{ U}:1 \text{ mL} = 16 \text{ U}:x \text{ mL}$$
$$100x = 16$$
$$x = {}^{16}\!/_{100}$$
$$x = 0.16 \text{ mL regular insulin}$$

$$100 \text{ U}:1 \text{ mL} = 30 \text{ U}:x \text{ mL}$$
$$100x = 30$$
$$x = {}^{30}\!/_{100}$$
$$x = 0.3 \text{ mL NPH insulin}$$

Answer: Total insulin needed is 0.46 mL (0.16 mL of regular insulin and 0.3 mL of NPH insulin). Using a tuberculin syringe, measure 0.16 mL of regular human insulin into the syringe and then fill to the 0.46 mark with NPH human insulin and administer every morning before breakfast. (Always measure the regular insulin first to avoid getting any of the NPH into the regular insulin vial.)

Problem 3: ORDERED: Novolin L insulin 80 U SC ac qAM
AVAILABLE: Human insulin zinc suspension (Novolin L) 100 U/mL and only 3 mL hypodermic syringes

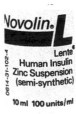

FIGURE 4–61 • Human insulin zinc suspension (Courtesy of Squibb-Nova, Inc.).

Solution:

$$100 \text{ U} : 16 \text{ m} = 80 \text{ U} : x \text{ m}$$
$$100x = 16 \times 80$$
$$100x = 1280$$
$$x = {}^{1280}\!/_{100}$$
$$x = 12.8 \text{ m}$$

Answer: A 3 mL syringe has no hundredths markings on it, so use 16 m = 1 mL in original equation. Using a 3 mL hypodermic syringe, draw up 12.8 m of Novolin N and give it before breakfast every day.

Practice Problems

Answers can be found in Appendix C, pp. 254–255.

Problem	Answer

1. ORDERED: Novolin N insulin 10 U 20 min ac qAM
   AVAILABLE: NPH human insulin isophane suspension (Novolin N) 100 U/mL, and no insulin syringe

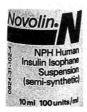

FIGURE 4–62 • NPH human insulin isophane suspension (Courtesy of Squibb-Nova, Inc.).

2. ORDERED: Novolin L insulin 18 U 1600 h qd
   AVAILABLE: Human insulin zinc suspension (Novolin L) 100 U/mL, and no insulin syringe

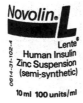

FIGURE 4–63 • Human insulin zinc suspension (Courtesy of Squibb-Nova, Inc.).

3. ORDERED: Novolin 70/30 95 U 1 h ac breakfast qd

Problem	**Answer**

AVAILABLE: 70% NPH human
insulin isophane suspension
and 30% regular human
insulin (Novolin 70/30), and
only a 3 mL syringe available

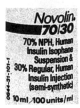

FIGURE 4–64 • 70% NPH human insulin isophane suspension and 30% regular human
insulin (Courtesy of Squibb-Nova, Inc.).

4. ORDERED: Novolin N 45 U and
   Novolin R 24 U 1 h ac
   breakfast tomorrow
   AVAILABLE: 100 U/mL NPH
   human insulin isophane
   suspension (Novolin N) and
   100 U/mL regular human
   insulin (Novolin R), and all
   insulin syringes

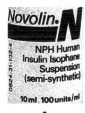 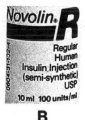

FIGURE 4–65 • NPH human insulin isophane
suspension and regular human insulin (Courtesy of Squibb-Nova, Inc.).

Read the insulin dosage indicated on each of the syringes shown here (assume all insulins are 100 U/mL):

Problem	**Answer**

5.

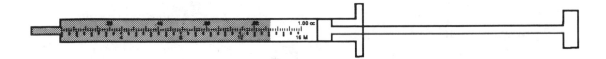

Problem	**Answer**

6.

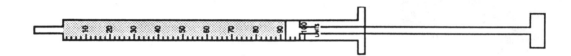

7.

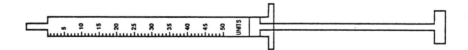

8.

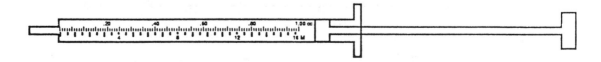

Mark the ordered dosage on the syringe provided for each problem.

9. Novolin 70/30 insulin 24 U

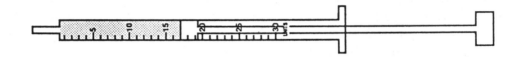

10. Novolin R insulin 15 U and
Novolin L insulin 30 U

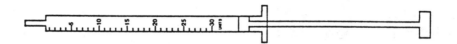

11. Novolin L insulin 75 U

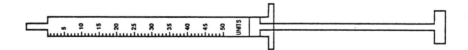

12. Novolin insulin 83 U

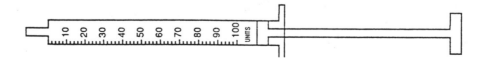

PART 16 • Intravenous Fluids and Medications

This is one of the most important sections of this book, first, because currently many drugs are given intravenously, and second, because an error in giving drugs intravenously is more serious than an error in giving drugs orally or by injection, when there is more time to take corrective action.

The equipment and supplies used to administer intravenous (IV) fluids and/or medications are so numerous and ever-changing that a complete explanation of these is beyond the scope of this book. However, some of these will be illustrated in a discussion designed to proceed from the simpler to the more complex IV solutions and drug problems.

RATE OF FLOW

When administering fluids intravenously, practitioners often must calculate and regulate the drops per minute in order to give a certain amount in the ordered period of time. The administration sets made by various manufacturers are constructed to yield varying numbers of drops per milliliter. This information can be found on the box containing the set. Examples of drops per milliliter are as follows:

10 gtts/mL—Baxter-Travenol
15 gtts/mL—Abbott
60 gtts/mL—Microdrip administration sets

The simplest type of IV problem involves the continuous administration of IV solutions without any medications added to the IV solution bag or bottle. IV fluids in bags will be used in all problems. Abbott is the only company that provides IV fluids in bottles. The connector is inserted into the primary solution container. The roller clamp ("FLO-TROL clamp" in Fig. 4–66, p. 141) is used to adjust the number of drops per minute of IV solution to be administered.

The steps in calculation of the number of drops per minute the IV should flow in order to give the desired amount in a specified time period are:

A. $\dfrac{\text{Total mL fluid to be given}}{\text{h to run}} = \text{Desired mL/h}$

B. $\text{Desired mL/h} \times \text{gtts/mL} = \text{Desired gtts/h}$

C. $\dfrac{\text{Desired gtts/h}}{60 \text{ min}} = \text{Desired gtts/min}$

Steps B and C can easily be reversed, as follows:

A. $\dfrac{\text{Total mL fluid to be given}}{\text{h to run}} = \text{Desired mL/h}$

B. $\dfrac{\text{Desired mL/h}}{60 \text{ min}} = \text{Desired mL/min}$

C. $\text{Desired mL/min} \times \text{gtts/mL} = \text{Desired gtts/min}$

Formula B can be used to calculate the regulation of flow of IV fluids as shown in Problem 1, Solutions 1 and 2, following. However, a much simpler method of calculation will be shown.

Example Problems

Problem 1: ORDERED: Give 1000 mL of 5% dextrose in water (D-5-W) IV in 2 h

AVAILABLE: Abbott administration set

Solution 1: FORMULA B: A, B, and C

A. $1000 \text{ mL} : 2 \text{ h} = x \text{ mL} : 1 \text{ h}$

$2x = 1000$

$x = {}^{1000}\!/_{2}$

$x = 500 \text{ mL/h}$

B. $1 \text{ mL} : 15 \text{ gtts} = 500 \text{ mL} : x \text{ gtts}$

$1x = 7500$

$x = 7500 \text{ gtts/h}$

C. $7500 \text{ gtts} : 60 \text{ min} = x \text{ gtts} : 1 \text{ min}$

$60x = 7500$

$x = {}^{7500}\!/_{60}$

$x = 125 \text{ gtts/min}$

Solution 2: FORMULA B: Steps B and C reversed

A. $1000 \text{ mL} : 2 \text{ h} = x \text{ mL} : 1 \text{ h}$

$2x = 1000$

$x = {}^{1000}\!/_{2}$

$x = 500 \text{ mL/h}$

B. $500 \text{ mL} : 60 \text{ min} = x \text{ mL} : 1 \text{ min}$

$60 \, x = 500$

$x = {}^{500}\!/_{60}$

$x = 8\tfrac{1}{3} \text{ mL/min}$

C. $1 \text{ mL} : 15 \text{ gtts} = 8\tfrac{1}{3} \text{ mL} : x \text{ gtts}$

$1x = {}^{25}\!/_{3} \times {}^{15}\!/_{1}$

$x = {}^{375}\!/_{3}$

$x = 125 \text{ gtts/min}$

Answer: Regulate IV to flow at 125 gtts/min initially to give 1000 mL D-5-W in 2 h.

Wherever practitioners work, they usually will be using only one manufacturer's IV administration sets. The simplified methods of calculating drops per minute are given here for Abbott's and Baxter-Travenol's regular (macrodrip) and microdrip (60 gtts/mL) sets.

A. Abbott set (15 gtts/mL):

$$\frac{\text{mL ordered}}{\text{h to run}} \times \frac{15}{60} = \frac{\text{mL ordered}}{\text{h to run}} \times \frac{1}{4} = \frac{\text{mL ordered}}{\text{h to run} \times 4} = \text{gtts/min}$$

or

$$\frac{\textbf{mL ordered}}{\textbf{h to run} \times 4} = \textbf{gtts/min}$$

B. Baxter-Travenol set (10 gtts/mL):

$$\frac{\text{mL ordered}}{\text{h to run}} \times \frac{10}{60} = \frac{\text{mL ordered}}{\text{h to run}} \times \frac{1}{6} = \frac{\text{mL ordered}}{\text{h to run} \times 6} = \text{gtts/min}$$

or

$$\frac{\textbf{mL ordered}}{\textbf{h to run} \times 6} = \textbf{gtts/min}$$

C. Abbott and Baxter-Travenol microdrip sets (60 gtts/mL):

$$\frac{\textbf{mL ordered}}{\textbf{h to run}} = \textbf{mL/h} = \textbf{gtts/min}$$

In Example A, directly above, one multiplies the milliliters per hour times 15 drops per mL and divides that amount by 60 minutes ($\frac{15}{60} = \frac{1}{4}$). In Example B, one multiplies the milliliters per hour times 10 drops per mL and divides that amount by 60 minutes ($\frac{10}{60} = \frac{1}{6}$). In Example C, the milliliters per hour equals the drops per minute by multiplying by 60 drops per mL and then dividing by 60 minutes.

Solution 3: Using the simplification of Formula B:

$$\frac{1000 \text{ mL}}{2 \text{ h} \times 4} = \frac{1000}{8} = 125 \text{ gtts/min,}$$

the same as in the previous Solutions 1 and 2.
Answer: Regulate the flow at 125 gtts/min initially.

Problem 2: ORDERED: 2000 mL of D-5-W by continuous drip qd
AVAILABLE: Baxter-Travenol administration set

Solution: $\dfrac{2000 \text{ mL}}{24 \text{ h} \times 6} = \dfrac{2000}{144} = 13.89 \text{ or } 14 \text{ gtts/min}$

Answer: Regulate IV at 14 gtts/min.

Practitioners should check the rate of flow of fluids at least every 30 minutes for patients whose IV sets are not connected to automatic flow control devices, and every hour otherwise. Other factors, such as the age and condition of the patient, may dictate the need for more frequent checks. It is not enough to count the drops per minute at these intervals because the fluid may have been running faster or slower than it should have been sometime during this interval. Therefore, every time one checks, after careful assessment of the patient's condition, speeding up or slowing down the IV may be indicated.

Calculated infusion flow rates are guidelines only. Maintaining the calculated rate of flow does not relieve health-care workers of their responsibility to observe for indications of too rapid or too slow an infusion. Fulfilling one's obligation to speed up, slow down, or stop an IV infusion at any time requires considerable judgment based upon many factors that are far beyond the scope of this book.

Problem 3: ORDERED: Give 1000 mL D-5-W in 2 h (When started at 0900 h, the IV was regulated to flow at 125 gtts/min; upon checking the IV bag at 0930 h, one finds 450 mL left in the bag)
AVAILABLE: Abbott administration set

Solution:

$$\frac{450 \text{ mL}}{1\frac{1}{2} \text{ h} \times 4} = \frac{450}{6} = 75 \text{ gtts/min}$$

Answer: At 0930 h regulate the flow of fluid at 75 gtts/min, or less, if indicated.

There was 450 mL left in the IV bag and 1½ hours left for it to run.
The IV infusion should be slowed to 75 drops per minute unless the patient's condition indicates that it should be given even slower, for a while at least.

Problem 4: ORDERED: 500 mL Ringer's lactate IV qd in 4 h
AVAILABLE: Microdrip (60 gtts/mL) administration set

Solution:

$$\frac{500 \text{ mL}}{4 \text{ h}} = 125 \text{ gtts/min}$$

Answer: Regulate the IV flow at 125 gtts/min.

Problem 5: ORDERED: 2000 mL D-5-W IV to run 24 h (When started at 1000 h, the IV was regulated to flow at 14 gtts/min–see Problem 2. Now it is 1200 h the same day, and 400 mL remain in the first 1000 mL bottle.)
AVAILABLE: Baxter-Travenol administration set

Solution:

$$\frac{400 \text{ mL}}{10 \text{ h} \times 6} = \frac{400}{60} = 6.67 \text{ or } 7 \text{ gtts/min}$$

Answer: Regulate the IV to flow at 7 gtts/min

The first 1000 mL was to run 12 hours, and 10 of those 12 hours remain.
Calculating on the basis of the 2000 mL in 24 hours would result in greater fluid infusion in the first 12 hours than during the second 12 hours. When starting the second 1000 mL, regulate the flow at 125 drops per minute again, as calculated in Problem 2.

Practice Problems

Answers can be found in Appendix C, pp. 255–256.

Problem	Answer
1. ORDERED: 1000 mL D-5-W IV in 4 h AVAILABLE: Baxter-Travenol administration set	

Problem	**Answer**
2. ORDERED: 1000 mL D-5-W to run IV at 250 mL/h AVAILABLE: Abbott administration set	
3. ORDERED: 1000 mL 0.45% sodium chloride, then 1000 mL D-5-W IV over 24 h AVAILABLE: Baxter-Travenol administration set	
4. ORDERED: 1500 mL D-5-W IV in 6 h today AVAILABLE: Baxter-Travenol administration set	
5. ORDERED: 1000 mL ½% sodium chloride then 2000 mL D-5-W IV to run 24 h AVAILABLE: Abbott administration set (IV infusion was started at 1000 h; at 1200 h there is 500 mL in the first bottle)	

Problem	**Answer**

6. ORDERED: Same as in Problem 5
   AVAILABLE: Same as in Problem
   5 (at 2200 h the same day 700
   mL remains in the second
   bottle)

7. ORDERED: Add 400 mL ⅙
   Ringer's lactate to IV, and run
   for 24 h
   AVAILABLE: Microdrip (60
   gtts/mL) administration set

8. ORDERED: 1000 mL D-10-W to
   run from 0900–1400 h today
   AVAILABLE: Baxter-Travenol
   administration set

9. ORDERED: 3000 mL D-5-W IV in
   24 h
   AVAILABLE: Abbott administration set

Problem	**Answer**

10. ORDERED: 1000 mL D-5-W IV at
    200 mL/h, then 500 mL ⅙
    Ringer's lactate at 100 mL/h
    AVAILABLE: Baxter-Travenol
    administration set

11. ORDERED: 1500 mL D-5-W IV in
    6 h
    AVAILABLE: Baxter-Travenol
    administration set

12. ORDERED: Run 1000 mL 0.45%
    sodium chloride at 200 mL/h
    for 1 h, then run at 50 mL/h
    AVAILABLE: Abbott administra-
    tion set

13. ORDERED: 500 mL D-10-W IV in
    4 h
    AVAILABLE: Abbott administra-
    tion set

Problem	Answer

14. ORDERED: 2000 mL D-5-W IV in
     10 h
     AVAILABLE: Abbott administra-
     tion set (IV started at 1530 h;
     at 1830 h there is 200 mL in
     the first bag)

15. ORDERED: 1000 mL D-5-W in
     3 h, then 500 mL 0.45%
     sodium chloride in 5 h
     AVAILABLE: Baxter-Travenol
     administration set (1000 mL
     D-5-W ran from 1000–1300 h;
     at 1400 h there is 250 mL in
     the 500 mL 0.45% sodium
     chloride bag)

INTRAVENOUS DRUGS BY INFUSION SETS

Primary Sets

Figure 4–66 is an example of a primary infusion set. Drugs are added to the IV fluid container according to the physicians's order.

Secondary Sets

Sometimes two IVs may be infusing at the same time, using what is called a secondary set (Fig. 4–67A). One or both of the IV containers may contain a medication. No problems of this kind are included here because each IV is prepared and regulated as a separate IV, using the control clamps above the point of the connection of the two tubings to regulate which one or two IVs will flow.

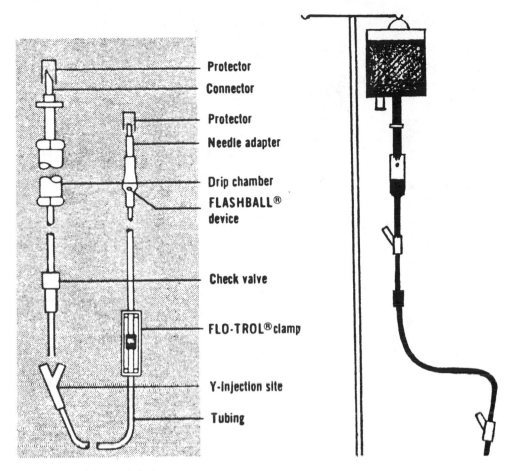

Protector
Connector
Protector
Needle adapter
Drip chamber
FLASHBALL® device
Check valve
FLO-TROL® clamp
Y-Injection site
Tubing

FIGURE 4–66 • Primary infusion set.

Add-a-Line Sets

Sometimes IV medications are added to a separate small volume IV fluid container and are given by a method commonly called add-a-line or piggy back (PB). The needle on these add-a-line units usually is inserted into a rubber-stoppered Y connector on the tubing of the main line IV tubing. In order for the fluid containing the medication to flow, this PB container must be elevated above the level of the main line IV fluid container (Fig. 4–67B). When the PB IV fluid bag is empty, the primary set will begin to flow at its preset rate.

Because these PB IV containers contain 50, 100, or 250 mL of fluid, this method is usually used for adults or older children only. Frequently the pharmacy adds the drug to the PB bag and properly labels the bags before they are sent to the nursing unit. However, on all units in most small hospitals and on some units in many large hospitals, practitioners still prepare all IV medication solutions.

Heparin Locks

Often IV medications are given via heparin locks, either by IV push from a syringe or in IV fluids given intermittently through a heparin lock (Fig. 4–68). The procedure used in most health-care agencies calls for the use of 2 to 5 mL of sterile isotonic saline

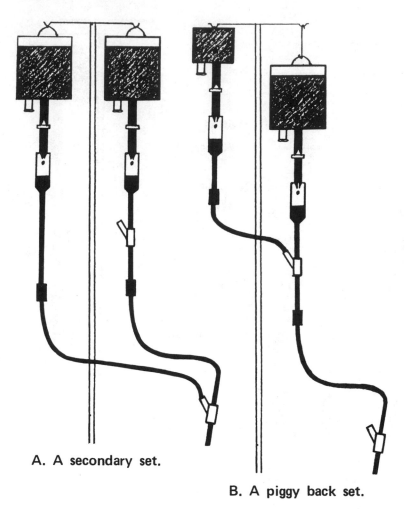

A. A secondary set.

B. A piggy back set.

FIGURE 4–67 • Two IV infusion methods **(A)** A secondary set. **(B)** A piggy back set.

to clear the heparin from the needle and intracath before administering the IV medication and the use of the same amount after giving the medication. Flushing the lock with sterile isotonic saline before and after giving the medication is especially important when the medication is incompatible with heparin.

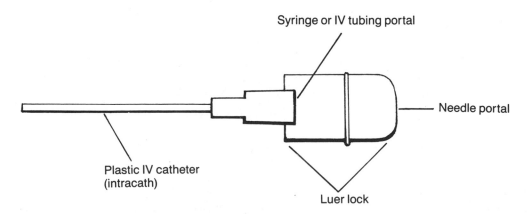

FIGURE 4–68 • Heparin lock.

Filling the needle and intracath with an ordered or indicated amount of heparin solution is the final step. The amount of heparin solution needed varies with the type of heparin lock used. For example, one kind needs 0.25 mL heparin as a flush, and another requires 0.6 mL. Special 1 mL heparin flush Tubex cartridges containing 10 or 100 U of heparin per mL usually are available for this purpose. If not, it may be necessary to dilute the available heparin to a weaker strength. Many hospitals now use sodium citrate instead of heparin to prevent occlusion of the heparin locks by clotting of the blood.

Example Problems:

Problem 1: ORDERED: 1000 mL D-5-W with 40 mEq KCl IV today at no more than 20 mEq/h

AVAILABLE: 10 mL vials of potassium chloride (KCl) containing 20 mEq of drug and Baxter-Travenol primary administration set

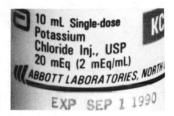

FIGURE 4–69 • Potassium chloride (From Abbott Laboratories with permission).

Solution: To prevent hyperkalemia no more than 10 to 40 mEq KCl/h (depending on serum potassium and patient's condition) should be given intravenously to adults

$$\frac{1000 \text{ mL}}{2 \text{ h} \times 6} = \frac{1000}{12} = 83\frac{1}{3} \text{ or } 83 \text{ gtts/min}$$

Answer: Add 20 mL (2 vials) of KCl to 1000 mL D-5-W. Regulate IV to flow at a maximum of 83 gtts/min initially.

Problem 2: ORDERED: Keep vein open (KVO) with D-5-W and Pipracil 4 g IV PB q4h

AVAILABLE: Piperacillin sodium (Pipracil) in 4 g vials; Baxter-Travenol primary and PB administration sets; and 50 and 100 mL PB solutions

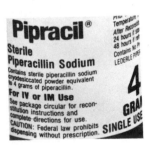

FIGURE 4–70 • Piperacillin sodium (From Lederle Laboratories with permission).

DIRECTIONS: Reconstitute each gram with 2 mL diluent to get 1 g/2.5 mL. For IV use, reconstitute drug with at least 5 mL/g and give over 3–5 min by IV push, or dilute further with at least 50 mL and give over 30 min.

Solution: Add a minimum of 8 mL diluent to a 4 g vial in order to dissolve the drug. Use a 12 mL syringe. There will be 10 mL of reconstituted solution.

$$1 \text{ g}:2.5 \text{ mL} = 4 \text{ g}:x \text{ mL}$$
$$1x = 10 \text{ mL}$$

A larger amount of diluent, up to the capacity of the vial, could be used. Add whatever amount of reconstituted drug is prepared to a 50 mL PB bag of an appropriate solution.

Adding 10 mL would result in a total of 60 mL, which the practitioner elects to run for 30 min

$$\frac{60 \text{ mL}}{\frac{1}{2} \text{ h} \times 6} = \frac{60}{3} = 20 \text{ gtts/min}$$

Answer: Add 8 mL of diluent to 4 g vial of Pipracil, add the resulting 10 mL of reconstituted drug to a 50 mL PB bag of solution, connect it to the primary set, elevate the PB above the primary set, and regulate the PB at 20 gtts/min. Leave primary set at KVO.

Problem 3: ORDERED: Clindamycin 500 mg IV q12h over 30 min by heparin lock. Use 100 U/mL heparin for lock.

AVAILABLE: Clindamycin phosphate (Cleocin) 600 mg (4 mL) vial; heparin 100 U in 1 mL Tubex syringes; IV PB fluid bags of 50, 100, and 250 mL each; and Abbott primary IV sets

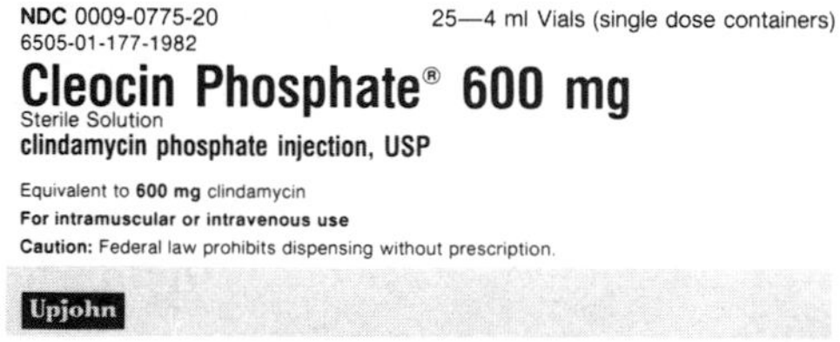

NDC 0009-0775-20   25—4 ml Vials (single dose containers)
6505-01-177-1982

Cleocin Phosphate® 600 mg
Sterile Solution
clindamycin phosphate injection, USP

Equivalent to **600 mg** clindamycin
For intramuscular or intravenous use
Caution: Federal law prohibits dispensing without prescription.

Upjohn

FIGURE 4–71 • Clindamycin phosphate (Courtesy of The Upjohn Company).

DIRECTIONS: Dilute to concentration no greater than 12 mg/mL and give no faster than 30 mg/min.

Solution:

$$600 \text{ mg}:4 \text{ mL} = 500 \text{ mg}:x \text{ mL}$$
$$600x = 2000$$
$$x = {}^{2000}\!/_{600}$$
$$x = 3.3 \text{ mL of drug}$$

$$12 \text{ mg}:1 \text{ mL} = 500 \text{ mg}:x \text{ mL}$$
$$12x = 500$$
$$x = {}^{500}\!/_{12}$$
$$x = 41.67 \text{ mL minimum fluid}$$

$$30 \text{ mg}:1 \text{ min} = 500 \text{ mg}:x \text{ min}$$
$$30x = 500$$
$$x = {}^{500}\!/_{30}$$
$$x = 16.67 \text{ min minimum time}$$

$$\frac{53 \text{ mL}}{\frac{1}{2} \text{ h} \times 4} \times \frac{53}{2} = 26.5 \text{ gtts/min}$$

Answer: Add 3.3 mL of clindamycin to a 50 mL PB bag of D-5-W, mix, and connect to IV tubing. Irrigate heparin lock with 2–5 mL of isotonic sterile saline and connect IV tubing to heparin lock. Regulate IV at 26–27 gtts/min. After IV has been given, irrigate heparin lock with 2–5 mL of isotonic saline. Then instill enough heparin 100 U/mL to fill the lock being used.

Practice Problems:

Answers can be found in Appendix C, pp. 256–257.

Problem	Answer

1. ORDERED: Primaxin 250 mg IV q6h and continuous D-5-0.45 NaCl at 40 mL/h

   AVAILABLE: Imipenem cilastatin sodium (Primaxin) 250 mg vials; 50, 100, and 250 mL PB bags of solution; and Abbott primary and secondary IV tubing sets (The practitioner decides to give drug in 30 min.)

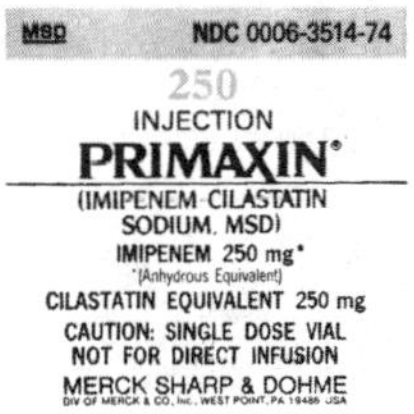

MSD   NDC 0006-3514-74
250
INJECTION
PRIMAXIN®
(IMIPENEM·CILASTATIN
SODIUM, MSD)
IMIPENEM 250 mg*
*(Anhydrous Equivalent)
CILASTATIN EQUIVALENT 250 mg
CAUTION: SINGLE DOSE VIAL
NOT FOR DIRECT INFUSION
MERCK SHARP & DOHME
DIV OF MERCK & CO., INC., WEST POINT, PA 19486 USA

FIGURE 4–72 • Imipenem-cilastatin sodium (Courtesy of Merck Sharp & Dohme).

   DIRECTIONS: Add 10 mL diluent to vial, dissolve drug, and add to 100 mL appropriate IV solution, and give over at least 20–30 min.

2. ORDERED: Kefzol 500 mg IV push q6h via heparin lock; use 10 U/mL heparin

   AVAILABLE: Cefazolin sodium (Kefzol) 500 mg vials for IV use

Problem	**Answer**

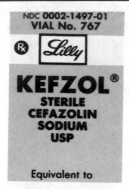

FIGURE 4–73 • Cefazolin sodium (Courtesy of Eli Lilly and Company).

DIRECTIONS: Dilute 500 mg in minimum of 10 mL sterile water for injection and inject slowly over 3–5 min. Irrigate lock before and after injection and instill heparin according to policy.

3. ORDERED: Primaxin 1 g IV q8h by intermittent PB IV and D-5-W running as KVO
AVAILABLE: Imipenem-cilastatin sodium (Primaxin) 500 mg vials; 100 mL PB IV solution; and Baxter-Travenol primary and PB IV administration sets

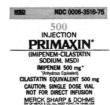

FIGURE 4–74 • Imipenem-cilastatin sodium (Courtesy of Merck Sharp & Dohme).

DIRECTIONS: Withdraw 10 mL from 100 mL appropriate IV solution bag to dissolve drug; add reconstituted drug to 100 mL bag; and give over 40–60

Problem	**Answer**

min. (The practitioner decides to give the drug in 60 min.)

4. ORDERED: Ticar 1 g IV q4h via heparin lock and intermittent drip

   AVAILABLE: Ticarcillin disodium (Ticar) 3 g ADD-Vantage vial; 50, 100, and 250 mL PB bags of IV solution; and Abbott primary IV set

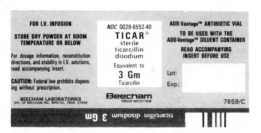

FIGURE 4–75 • Ticarcillin disodium (Courtesy of Beecham Laboratories).

   DIRECTIONS: Dissolve drug as directed and dilute to between 10 and 100 mg/mL. Give over 30 min.

5. ORDERED: Unasyn 1.5 g IV q6h via heparin lock

   AVAILABLE: Ampicillin sodium/subactum sodium (Unasyn) 1.5 g vial; 50, 100, and 250 mL PB bags of appropriate IV solutions; and Abbott primary administration set

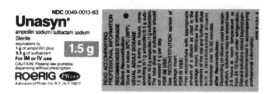

FIGURE 4–76 • Ampicillin sodium/subactam sodium (Courtesy of Roerig).

Problem   **Answer**

DIRECTIONS: Diluting 1.5 g vial
of ampicillin sodium/subactum
sodium with 3.2 mL of sterile
water yields 4 mL of
reconstituted drug. Further
dilute the drug in 50–100 mL
of a compatible solution and
give over 15–30 min.

6. ORDERED: Gentamicin 70 mg IV
q8h PB and KVO with D-5-W
AVAILABLE: Gentamicin sulfate
in 80 mg in 2 mL Dosette
vials; 50, 100, and 250 mL
bags of D-5-W and isotonic
saline; and Baxter-Travenol
primary and secondary IV sets

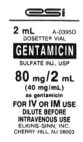

FIGURE 4–77 • Gentamicin sulfate (Courtesy
of Elkins-Sinn, Inc.).

DIRECTIONS: Dilute single dose
in 50–200 mL of isotonic
saline or D-5-W and infuse
over ½–2 h.

7. ORDERED: Aminophylline 250
mg very slowly by IV push
via heparin lock stat
AVAILABLE: Anhydrous
theophylline 19.7 mg/mL and
ethylenediamine 3.69 mg/mL
(aminophylline 25 mg/mL) in
10 mL vial

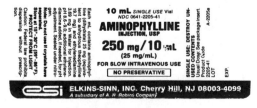

FIGURE 4–78 • Aminophylline (Courtesy of
Elkins-Sinn, Inc.).

Problem	Answer

DIRECTIONS: Do not exceed rate
of 25 mg/min.

8. ORDERED: Penicillin G potassium
5,000,000 U in continuous IV
of 1000 mL D-5-W q12h
AVAILABLE: Penicillin G
potassium (Pfizerpen) in
5,000,000 U 20 mL vial and
Abbott primary administration
set

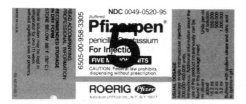

FIGURE 4–79 • Penicillin G potassium (Courtesy of Roerig).

DIRECTIONS:

DILUENT	U/ML
18.2 mL	250,000
8.2 mL	500,000
3.2 mL	1,000,000

9. ORDERED: Heparin 5000 U IV
injection stat followed by
30,000 U/24h in 1000 mL
0.45% sodium chloride
AVAILABLE: Heparin 10,000
U/mL in 4 mL multiple dose
vial; Baxter-Travenol primary
administration set; and 1000
mL bags of 0.45% sodium
chloride

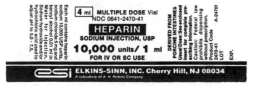

FIGURE 4–80 • Heparin sodium (Courtesy of Elkins-Sinn, Inc.).

DIRECTIONS: After adding
heparin to a continuous IV
infusion solution, invert the

Problem	**Answer**

container at least six times to
ensure adequate mixing.

10. ORDERED: Diphenhydramine 100
     mg in 50 mL D-5-W IV PB
     stat over 15 min, then 50 mg
     in 50 mL D-5-W IV PB q4h
     over 30 min and KVO with
     D-5-W
   AVAILABLE: Diphenhydramine
     hydrochloride 50 mg/mL in 1
     mL Dosette vials; 50 mL bags
     of D-5-W; and Baxter-
     Travenol administration set

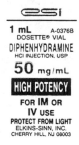

FIGURE 4–81 • Diphenhydramine hydrochloride (Courtesy of Elkins-Sinn, Inc.).

DIRECTIONS: Dosage should be
     individualized according to the
     needs and the response of the
     patient.

PART 17 • Intravenous Therapy by Controlled Mechanisms

Many machines available today automatically regulate the flow of IV solutions at the rate to which they are set. These machines are almost always used for infants and small children and frequently for older children and adults. With them it is possible to maintain very slow rates of flow. However, very close observation of pediatric and adult patients receiving intravenous fluid for indications of too rapid or too slow infusion rates is imperative.

Intravenous flow regulation machines can be classified into three general types: automatic controllers, volume delivery pumps, and syringe infusers. Although some of the capabilities of these machines will be given, the emphasis in the example and the practice problems will be on the correct dosage, the concentration of the drug, and the correct rate of flow.

AUTOMATIC CONTROLLERS

The automatic controllers, such as IVACs 230 and 260, regulate the flow rate by drops per minute according to the drop size of the administration set being used. These machines *do not* exert pressure on the fluid being infused, and the actual flow rate may vary at times from the rate at which the machines are set. The flow rate can be affected by the position of the patient, the IV fluid container, and/or the IV tubing, and by the size of the venipuncture needle or catheter. Because of this, these machines are being replaced by infusion machines that *do* exert pressure.

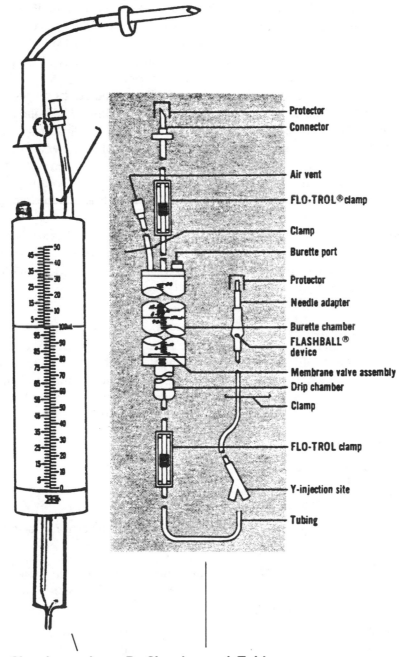

A. Chamber only.   B. Chamber and Tubing.

FIGURE 4–82 • Fluid volume control chamber. **(A)** Chamber only. **(B)** Chamber and tubing.

Usually a fluid volume control chamber or burette, for example, a Buretrol or a Soluset, is used with these machines. These chambers hold 100 or 150 mL and have a calibrated mark for each 2 mL. Most often these chambers have microdrip (60 gtts/mL) inlets. If a microdrip set is used, a machine set to deliver 20 drops per minute should deliver 20 mL per hour.

In most instances, the clamp above the chamber is opened and an hour's supply of fluid is added to the 5 or 10 mL residual fluid that is to be left in the chamber at the end of each hour in order to prevent air from getting into the tubing below. Limiting the amount of fluid that can be infused to an hour's supply is an added precaution against fluid overload.

Medications may be put into the rubber-stoppered inlet (Burette Port in Fig. 4-82) on the fluid volume chambers with a syringe and needle or with a secondary IV PB set (Fig. 4-67B). Then the indicated amount of IV fluid is added from the primary fluid bag or from the PB bag. Medications also can be injected into any of the portals on the IV tubing below the pump. This is discussed farther on.

A general rule, especially for infants and children and adults on restricted fluids, is to infuse drugs at the same rate as the continuous IV fluid. The hourly milliliter intake should not be increased appreciably as a result of the medications.

Although 5 or 10 mL should be left in volume control chambers at the end of each hour when giving the primary IV fluid, after a medication has been added to the chamber it should be emptied completely before adding another hour's supply (plus 5 or 10 mL) to the chamber. This requires close observation so that air does not get into the tubing as the chamber is emptying.

Whenever a drug is added to an IV system, a label should be placed on the IV bag, the volume control chamber, or the infuser pump syringe containing the medication. On the label, write the name and amount of the drug and the time it was added. Remove the label when the drug has infused completely.

Example Problems:

Problem 1: ORDERED: Pentam 200 mg IV qd and D-5-W at 35 mL/h

AVAILABLE: Pentamidine isethionate (Pentam), 300 mg single dose vial; IVAC 230 controller with microdrip burette; and 50, 100, and 250 mL PB bags of solution.

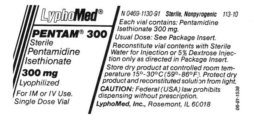

FIGURE 4-83 • Pentamidine isethionate (Courtesy of LyphoMed, Inc.).

DIRECTIONS: Give adults and children 4 mg/kg once a day. Dissolve the contents of the vial in 3 mL of sterile water, dilute further in 50-250 mL of D-5-W, and infuse over 60 min.

Solution: $300 \text{ mg} : 3 \text{ mL} = 200 \text{ mg} : x \text{ mL}$

$$300x = 600$$
$$x = {}^{600}\!/_{300}$$
$$x = 2 \text{ mL}$$

Answer: At the end of the hour, there should be 10 mL of the primary IV solution in the burette, according to the hospital policy. The 2 mL of drug could be added to the burette and 48 mL of the D-5-W could be added to bring the total in the burette to 50 mL. Increase the flow to 50 gtts/min (50 mL/h). Let the burette empty at the end of the hour before adding 45 mL (35 mL for the next hour and 10 mL reserve) of D-5-W. Resume flow at 35 gtts/min (35 mL/h).

Problem 2: ORDERED: Polycillin-N 125 mg IV q6h and D-5-W at 40 mL/h
AVAILABLE: Ampicillin sodium (Polycillin-N) 125 mg vial; IVAC 260 controller; a microdrip burette; and 500 mL bag of D-5-W

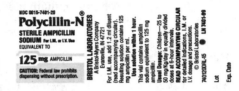

FIGURE 4–84 • Ampicillin sodium (Courtesy of Bristol Laboratories).

DIRECTIONS: Add 1.2 mL diluent to get 125 mg/mL. Dilute to 2–30 mg/mL for IV use and give within 4 h.

Solution:
$$30 \text{ mg} : 1 \text{ mL} = 125 \text{ mg} : x \text{ mL}$$
$$30x = 125$$
$$x = {}^{125}\!/_{30}$$
$$x = 4.167 \text{ mL minimum fluid}$$
$$2 \text{ mg} : 1 \text{ mL} = 125 \text{ mg} : x \text{ mL}$$
$$2x = 125$$
$$x = {}^{125}\!/_{2}$$
$$x = 62.5 \text{ mL maximum fluid}$$

Answer: At the end of the hour, there would be 10 mL of the D-5-W left in the burette, according to hospital policy. Add 1.2 mL diluent to the 125 mg drug vial and withdraw 1 mL. Add the 1 mL of drug to the burette, and fill the burette to 40 mL and continue flow at 40 gtts/min (40 mL/h). Let the burette empty at the end of the hour, then add 50 mL D-5-W and regulate the flow at 40 gtts/min.

Problem 3: ORDERED: Gentamicin 30 mg IV q8h over 1 h and 50 mL D-5-W per h to an 18-month-old child
AVAILABLE: Gentamicin sulfate 20 mg/2 mL; IVAC 230 controller; a 150 mL microdrip burette; and 500 mL bags of D-5-W

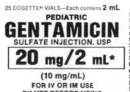

FIGURE 4–85 • Gentamicin sulfate (Courtesy of Elkins-Sinn, Inc.).

DIRECTIONS: Dosage for children with normal renal function is 6–7.5 mg/kg/day. Dilute in isotonic saline or D-5-W before administering. Do not mix with other drugs. Infuse over ½–2 h.

Solution:
$$20 \text{ mg}:2 \text{ mL} = 30 \text{ mg}:x \text{ mL}$$
$$20x = 60$$
$$x = 3 \text{ mL}$$

Answer: Add 3 mL of gentamicin to the 10 mL of D-5-W remaining in the burette at the end of the hour. Add 40 mL D-5-W to the burette. Continue the flow at 50 gtts/min (mL/h = gtts/min). Let the burette empty completely at the end of the hour (to ensure administration of all of the drug); then add 60 mL (50 mL/h plus 10 mL reserve).

Practice Problems

Answers can be found in Appendix C, pp. 257–258.

Problem	Answer

1. ORDERED: Staphcillin 1 g IV q6h and Ringer's lactate at 15 mL/h
   AVAILABLE: Methicillin sodium (Staphcillin), 4 g vial, and IVAC 230 automatic controller with macrodrip burette (10 gtts/mL); hospital policy calls for 10 mL IV fluid reserve in burette at the end of each hour

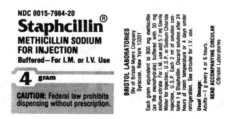

FIGURE 4–86 • Methicillin sodium (Courtesy of Bristol Laboratories).

DIRECTIONS: Add 5.7 mL diluent to 4 g vial to get 1 g/2 mL of reconstituted drug. May put 1 g in 50 mL of appropriate IV solution and give at 10 mL/min or dilute drug to concentrations of 10–30 mg/mL.

2. ORDERED: Decadron 1 mg IV q12h and D-5-0.45 NaCl continuous IV via IVAC 260 automatic controller, at 30 mL/h via macrodrip burette

Problem	**Answer**

AVAILABLE: Dexamethasone
sodium (Decadron) 4 mg/mL in
1 mL vial; macrodrip (15
gtts/mL) IV burette; and 250,
500, and 1000 mL bags of
D-5-0.45 NaCl

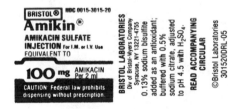

FIGURE   4–87 • Dexamethasone   sodium
(Courtesy of Merck Sharp & Dohme).

DIRECTIONS: For IV drip add drug
to NaCl or dextrose solutions.

3.   ORDERED: Amikin 100 mg IV
q8h and D-5-0.2 NaCl at 30
mL/h
AVAILABLE: Amikacin sulfate
(Amikin) 100 mg/2 mL vial;
microdrip burette; and IVAC
230 automatic controller

FIGURE 4–88 • Amikacin sulfate (Courtesy of
Bristol Laboratories).

DIRECTIONS: Add 0.5 g to 100–
200 mL IV fluid. For children,
use enough diluent to give
over 30–60 min. For infants
use enough diluent to give
over 1–2 h. Give at same rate
as IV is running, if possible.
(The practitioner decides to run
the fluid with the drug for 1 h.)

4.   ORDERED: Primaxin 250 mg IV
q6h and KVO at 5 mL/h with
D-5-W
AVAILABLE: Imipenem-cilastatin
sodium (Primaxin) 250 mg

Problem	**Answer**

vials; macrodrip (15 gtts/mL) burette; 1000 mL bags of D-5-W; and IVAC 230 controller

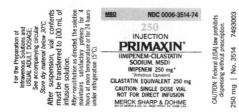

FIGURE 4–89 • Imipenem-cilastatin sodium (Courtesy of Merck Sharp & Dohme).

DIRECTIONS: Add 10 mL of diluent to vial and agitate until clear. Dilute further in 100 mL of appropriate diluent. Give 250 mg or 500 mg dose IV over 20–30 min and a 1000 mg dose over 40–60 min.

5. ORDERED: Gentamicin 120 mg IV q8h and D-5-W at 100 mL/h
    AVAILABLE: Gentamicin sulfate 80 mg/2 mL Dosette vials; macrodrip (10 gtts/mL) burette; 50, 100, 250, and 1000 mL bags of D-5-W; and IVAC 260 controller

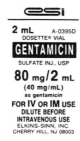

FIGURE 4–90 • Gentamicin sulfate (Courtesy of Elkins-Sinn, Inc.).

DIRECTIONS: For intermittent IV infusion to adults, dilute drug in 50 to 200 mL isotonic saline or 5% dextrose and infuse over ½–2 h. Do not mix with other drugs.

VOLUME DELIVERY PUMPS

The fluid volume delivery pumps are the second general type of IV infusion machine. These *do* exert a pressure on the infusing fluid; therefore, the flow volume remains constant. They control the milliliters per hour at the amount to which they are set. Some can be set to 0.1 mL per hour. Either microdrip or macrodrip fluid volume chambers and other administration sets may be used with these machines. Most machines require the use of the company's own primary, secondary, piggy back (PB), multiple Y, burette, or check valve administrations sets. There is one machine that will accommodate six IV tubings at once. Medications may be introduced into any of the portals in the particular IV system. Most volume delivery pumps have alarm systems providing as many as 12 messages of alarm-action problems due to any occlusion–clogged filter, closed tubing clamp, clogged airway to IV bag, and the like.

Teaching one how to use these machines is far beyond the scope of this book; however, to illustrate the phenomenal capabilities of the machines, some examples follow:

- LIFECARE 5000 PLUM infusion system (Abbott)
  - will accommodate single fluid, PB, and multidose regimens with primary and secondary sets concurrently
  - can be used for blood administration and enteral feedings
  - can deliver from 1 to 999.9 mL/h with a maximum of 9999 mL with macrodrip primary, secondary, and multidose settings
  - can deliver from 0.1 to 99.9 mL/h with a maximum of 999 mL with microdrip primary, secondary, and multidose settings
  - can deliver from 2 to 24 secondary medication doses every 15 minutes for 24 hours with macrodrip and microdip settings
  - can be adjusted with pressure from 0.1 to 8 pounds per square inch (psi)
- LIFE CARE 4100 PCA PLUS infuser (Abbott)
  - in the PCA mode, administers drug upon patient demand with a 4 hour dose limit
  - in continuous mode, administers medication at a continuous rate with a 4 hour dose limit
  - in PCA and continuous modes, delivers a continuous dose plus patient-controller supplementary doses
  - has a lockout interval from 5 to 100 minutes in 1 minute increments
- PCA PUMP (BARD)
  - delivers continuous or patient regulated infusions at 0.1 to 99.9 mL/h in 0.1 mL/h increments
  - has automatic KVO at 0.5 mL/h
- imed 960 Volumetric Infusion Pump (IMED)
  - delivers 1 to 200 mL/h with maximum of 9999 mL, but 2 to 3 mL/h needed to KVO
- imed 927 Volumetric Infusion Pump (IMED)
  - delivers from 0.1 to 299 mL/h and maximum of 999 mL
- imed 965 Microvolumetric Infusion Pump (IMED)
  - delivers from 0.1 to 99.9 mL/h and maximum of 999.9 mL
- IVAC 530 infuser (IVAC)
  - delivers drops per minute according to pump flow conversion chart up to a maximum of 200 mL/h at 40 psi and are, therefore, used only in hyperbaric chambers
- AVI 400 A Volumetric Infusion Pump (3 M)
  - used with AVI Checkvalve Administration Set can, in 1 mL/h increments, switch automatically from PB rate and volume to different primary rate and volume of from 1 to 999 mL/h in 1 mL increments

- AVI Micro 275 Volumetric Pump (3 M)
  - keeps vein open at 1 mL/h automatically, or at less than 1 mL/h when set to do so
  - can run PB at different rate at maximum of 99.9 mL/h
- AVI 100, Micro 110, 200 A, Micro 210 A, 400 A, 270, 470, and Micro 275 (3M) are additional examples of some of the other machines available

Example Problems

Problem 1: ORDERED: D-5-W at 5 mL/h and give Mannitol 12.5 g IV, q3h in 30 min, if urinary output falls below 30 mL/h in previous hour(s)

AVAILABLE: Mannitol 25% (12.5 g/50 mL) in 50 mL vial, and imed 960 Volumetric Infusion Pump with 150 mL macrodrip burette (15 gtts/mL)

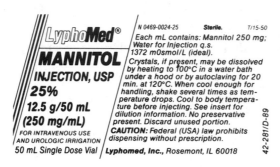

FIGURE 4–91 • Mannitol (Courtesy of Lypho-Med, Inc.).

DIRECTIONS: No special directions given.

Solution: No calculation is necessary.

Answer: Put the 50 mL of 25% Mannitol in the burette, which has 10 mL residual fluid at the end of each hour. Regulate the 60 mL to flow at 120 mL/h. When burette is empty at the end of 30 min, add 15 mL of D-5-W (5 mL/h plus 10 mL reserve).

Problem 2: ORDERED: Aminophyllin 8 mg/h continuous IV in D-5-W q24h

AVAILABLE: Aminophylline (Aminophyllin) 250 mg/10 mL vial, imed 960 Volumetric Infusion Pump, and 50, 100, and 250 mL IV PB bags of D-5-W.

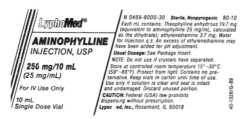

FIGURE 4–92 • Aminophylline (Courtesy of LyphoMed, Inc.).

DIRECTIONS: May add to 100–200 mL of appropriate IV fluid. Aminophylline is incompatible with many drugs, so flush the IV line between giving aminophylline and other drugs.

Solution:
$$8 \text{ mg}:1 \text{ h} = x \text{ mg}:24 \text{ h}$$
$$x = 192 \text{ mg of drug/24 h}$$

$$1 \text{ mg}:1 \text{ mL} = 192 \text{ mg}:x \text{ mL}$$
$$x = 192 \text{ mL is minimum fluid needed}$$

$$250 \text{ mg}:250 \text{ mL} = 8 \text{ mg}:x \text{ mL}$$
$$250x = 2000$$
$$x = {}^{2000}\!/_{250}$$
$$x = 8 \text{ mL/h is rate of flow}$$

Answer: Add 10 mL vial containing aminophylline 250 mg to a 250 mL PB bag, attach to imed machine, and set rate at 8 mL/h.

Problem 3: ORDERED: Nitropress 300 mcg/min IV for 5 min stat, then titrate dose to blood pressure, plus KVO with D-5-W

AVAILABLE: Sodium nitroprusside (Nitropress) 50 mg vial; LIFE-CARE 5000 PLUM infusion system with microdrip primary and secondary administration sets; and 250, 500, and 1000 mL bags of D-5-W

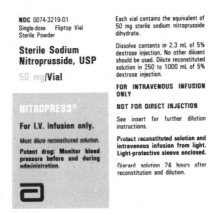

FIGURE 4–93 • Sodium nitroprusside (Courtesy of Abbott Laboratories).

DIRECTIONS: Dissolve drug in 2.3 mL of D-5-W; no other diluent should be used. Each 2 mL of reconstituted solution will contain 50 mg of the drug, which should be diluted further in 250–1000 mL of D-5-W. Promptly cover IV bag with drug and IV tubing with aluminum foil or other opaque material to protect from light.

Solution: Add 2 mL (50 mg) reconstituted drug to 250 mL of D-5-W.

$$50 \text{ mg}:250 \text{ mL} = 0.3 \text{ mg (300 mcg ordered)}:x \text{ mL}$$
$$50x = 75$$
$$x = 1.5 \text{ mL/min or 90 mL/h}$$

Answer: Start primary IV of D-5-W and set at KVO rate. Add 2.3 mL of D-5-W to 50 mg vial; add 2 mL of reconstituted drug to 250 mL of D-5-W; protect bag and secondary administration set tubing from light; regulate volume delivery pump to deliver 90 mL/h via secondary set for 5 min, checking blood pressure frequently. Then regulate infusion of drug as indicated by blood pressure readings.

Problem 4: ORDERED: Start D-5-W stat at 5 mL/h and give epinephrine IV push according to emergency room guidelines to a 33 lb child, and repeat q5–10 min as indicated by electrocardiogram readings.

AVAILABLE: Epinephrine 1:10,000 in 10 mL Abboject syringe; 250 mL bags of D-5-W; and AVI micro 275 Volumetric Pump

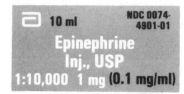

FIGURE 4–94 • Epinephrine (Courtesy of Elkins-Sinn, Inc.).

DIRECTIONS: Emergency room standing order guidelines are "to give 0.01 mg/kg or 0.1 mL/kg of 1:10,000 epinephrine by IV push." Hospital policy calls for injecting IV push medications into the IV tubing portal nearest the venipuncture site.

Solution:

$$0.01 \text{ mg}:1 \text{ kg} = x \text{ mg}:15 \text{ kg (33 lb)}$$
$$1x = 0.15 \text{ mg to be given}$$

$$1:10,000 = 1 \text{ g}:10,000 \text{ mL}$$
$$= 1000 \text{ mg}:10,000 \text{ mL}$$
$$= 1 \text{ mg}:10 \text{ mL}$$
$$= 0.1 \text{ mg}:1 \text{ mL}$$

$$0.1 \text{ mg}:1 \text{ mL} = 0.15 \text{ mg}:x \text{ mL}$$
$$0.1x = 0.15$$
$$x = 1.5 \text{ mL to be given}$$

Answer: Start IV with 250 mL of D-5-W; regulate volume delivery pump at 5 mL/h; inject 1.5 mL of 1:10,000 epinephrine into the flashball immediately; and give 1.5 mL q5–10 min as indicated by electrocardiogram readings.

Problem 5: ORDERED: Aminophyllin 50 mg IV PB in 1 h, 10 mg/h next 12 h, then 8 mg/h to 1-year-old child and D-5-W at 40 mL/h

AVAILABLE: Theophylline (Aminophyllin) 80 mg/100 mL in 500 mL D-5-W IV bag; AVI 400 A Volumetric Infusion Pump; and 1000 mL bag of D-5-W

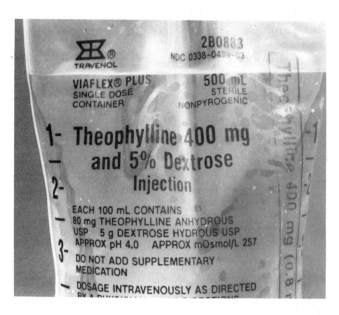

FIGURE 4–95 • Theophylline (From Travenol Laboratories, Inc. with permission).

DIRECTIONS: Do not give loading dose of drug faster than 25 mg/min. Theophylline is incompatible with many drugs.

Solution:
$$80 \text{ mg} : 100 \text{ mL } (1:1) = 50 \text{ mg} : x \text{ mL}$$
$$80x = 5000 \text{ mL}$$
$$x = {}^{5000}\!/_{80}$$
$$x = 62.5 \text{ mL}$$

$$80 \text{ mg} : 100 \text{ mL} = 10 \text{ mg} : x \text{ mL}$$
$$80x = 1000 \text{ mL}$$
$$x = {}^{1000}\!/_{80}$$
$$x = 12.5 \text{ mL}$$

$$80 \text{ mg} : 100 \text{ mL} = 8 \text{ mg} : x \text{ mL}$$
$$80x = 800$$
$$x = {}^{800}\!/_{80}$$
$$x = 10 \text{ mL}$$

Answer: Regulate primary D-5-W fluid at 40 mL/h. Using 80 mg/100 mL theophylline 500 mL PB bag, regulate volume delivery pump PB rate at 62.5 mL/h for 1 h; 12.5 mL/h for the next 12 h; then 10 mL/h.

Problem 6: ORDERED: Mefoxin 375 mg IV q6h to a 1-year-old child at same rate as D-5-W at 40 mL/h

AVAILABLE: Cefoxitin sodium (Mefoxin) 1 g vial; 50 mL bag of D-5-W; and imed 927 Volumetric Infusion Pump

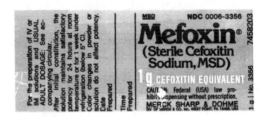

FIGURE 4–96 • Cefoxitin sodium (Courtesy of Merck Sharp & Dohme).

DIRECTIONS: Reconstitute 1 g with at least 10 mL of sterile water. Adding 10 mL of diluent will yield 10.5 mL of drug solution containing approximately 95 mg/mL.

Solution: Add 10 mL sterile water to 1 g vial of drug, and mix.

$$95 \text{ mg} : 1 \text{ mL} = 375 \text{ mg} : x \text{ mL}$$
$$95x = 375$$
$$x = {}^{375}\!/_{95}$$
$$x = 3.9 \text{ mL}$$

Answer: Withdraw 3.9 mL of reconstituted drug and add it to a 50 mL bag of D-5-W, mix, and administer via volume delivery pump at 40 mL/h for 1¼ h (40 mL:1 h = 54 mL:x h). When infused, add plain D-5-W and run at 40 mL/h.

Practice Problems

Answers can be found in Appendix C, pp. 258–259.

Problem	Answer

1. ORDERED: Primaxin 500 mg IV q6h and D-5-0.45 NaCl continuous IV running at 50 mL/h

   AVAILABLE: Imipenem-cilastatin sodium (Primaxin) 500 mg vial; AVI 400A Volumetric Infusion Pump; all sizes of PB fluids

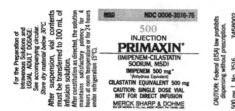

FIGURE 4–97 • Imipenem-cilastatin sodium (Courtesy of Merck Sharp & Dohme).

   DIRECTIONS: Dilute 250 mg or 500 mg in 100 mL of IV fluid. Withdraw 10 mL from the 100 mL IV bag, add this to the drug vial, mix, withdraw the drug solution, and add the appropriate amount back into the IV bag. Give 250–500 mg IV over at least 20–30 min; slow IV if nausea occurs.

2. ORDERED: Aminophyllin 30 mg/h continuous IV with 500 mg in 500 mL D-5-W

   AVAILABLE: Aminophylline (Aminophyllin) 500 mg/20 mL ampule; imed 927 Volumetric Infusion Pump; and 500 mL bags of D-5-W.

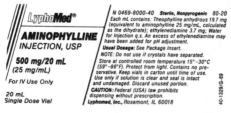

FIGURE 4–98 • Aminophylline (Courtesy of LyphoMed, Inc.).

Problem	Answer

DIRECTIONS: Drug may be injected slowly by syringe, not to exceed 25 mg/min, or 250 or 500 mg may be put in 100–200 mL.

3. ORDERED: Neo-Synephrine 40 mcg/min continuous IV in D-5-W

   AVAILABLE: Phenylephrine hydrochloride (Neo-Synephrine) 1% (10 mg/mL) in 1 mL ampules and imed 927 Volumetric Infusion Pump (Practitioner decides to put 10 mg in 500 mL of D-5-W.)

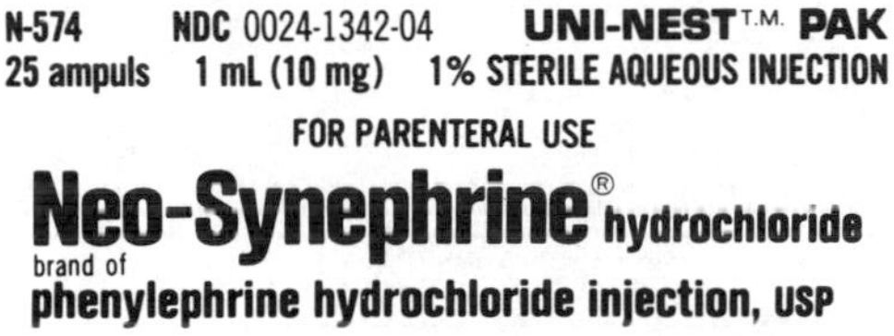

N-574   NDC 0024-1342-04   **UNI-NEST**™ **PAK**
25 ampuls   1 mL (10 mg)   1% STERILE AQUEOUS INJECTION
FOR PARENTERAL USE

Neo-Synephrine® hydrochloride
brand of
phenylephrine hydrochloride injection, USP

FIGURE 4–99 • Phenylephrine hydrochloride (Courtesy of Winthrop Pharmaceuticals).

DIRECTIONS: Adding 10 mg to 500 mL yields a 1:50,000 solution.

4. ORDERED: Septra 50 mg IV q8h and IV of D-5-W at KVO with AVI Micro 275 Volumetric Infusion Pump

   AVAILABLE: Trimethoprim and sulfamethoxazole (Septra) and 50, 100, and 250 mL IV PB bags of D-5-W. Each 5 mL vial contains 80 mg t(16 mg/mL) and 400 mg s(80 mg/mL). Amount ordered is based on t component of the drug.

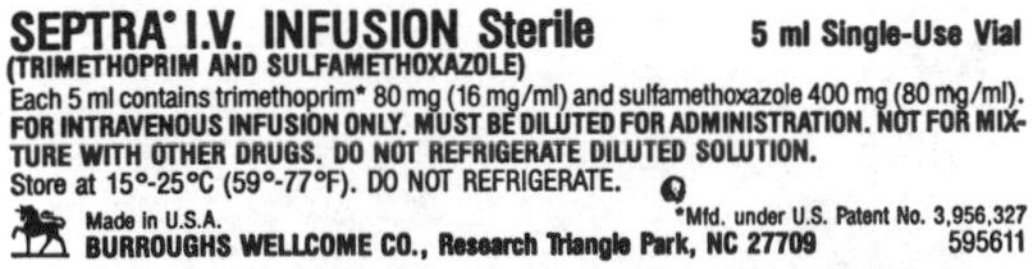

SEPTRA® I.V. INFUSION Sterile   5 ml Single-Use Vial
(TRIMETHOPRIM AND SULFAMETHOXAZOLE)
Each 5 ml contains trimethoprim* 80 mg (16 mg/ml) and sulfamethoxazole 400 mg (80 mg/ml).
FOR INTRAVENOUS INFUSION ONLY. MUST BE DILUTED FOR ADMINISTRATION. NOT FOR MIXTURE WITH OTHER DRUGS. DO NOT REFRIGERATE DILUTED SOLUTION.
Store at 15°-25°C (59°-77°F). DO NOT REFRIGERATE.
Made in U.S.A.   *Mfd. under U.S. Patent No. 3,956,327
BURROUGHS WELLCOME CO., Research Triangle Park, NC 27709   595611

FIGURE 4–100 • Trimethoprim and sulfamethoxazole (Courtesy of Burroughs Wellcome Co.).

Problem	**Answer**

DIRECTIONS: Mix with D-5-W
only. No rapid or bolus
injection. Each 5 mL vial
should be added to 125 mL of
D-5-W or as little as 75 mL, if
patient is to receive restricted
fluids. Give over 60–90 min.
Do not refrigerate. Use within
6 h. (The practitioner decides
to give the medicine in 60
min.)

5. ORDERED: Na bicarb 1 mEq/h for
24 h in D-5-W at 12 mL/h to
3 kg neonate
AVAILABLE: Infant 4.2% sodium
bicarbonate 5 mEq in 10 mL
syringe; imed 927 Volumetric
Infusion Pump; and 50 mL
bag of D-5-W

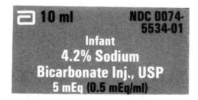

FIGURE 4–101 • Sodium bicarbonate (Courtesy of Abbott Laboratories).

DIRECTIONS: No special
directions given.

6. ORDERED: Dopamine at 150
mcg/min initially in 250 mL
D-5-W
AVAILABLE: Dopamine 200 mg
in 5 mL ampules; 250 mL of
D-5-W; and imed 965
Microvolumetric Infusion
Pump

FIGURE 4–102 • Dopamine hydrochloride (Courtesy of Elkins-Sinn, Inc.).

Problem	**Answer**

DIRECTIONS: Add 200 or 400 mg to 250 or 500 mL, respectively, of appropriate IV fluid before infusing. Closely observe vital signs and urinary output.

7. ORDERED: Gentamicin 70 mg IV q8h and D-5-W at 200 mL/h
   AVAILABLE: Gentamicin sulfate 80 mg/2 mL in 2 mL Dosette vials; 50, 100, 250, and 1000 mL bags of D-5-W; and AVI 400 A Volumetric Infusion Pump

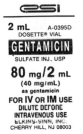

esi

2 mL   A-0395D
DOSETTE® VIAL
GENTAMICIN
SULFATE INJ., USP
80 mg/2 mL
(40 mg/mL)
as gentamicin
FOR **IV** OR **IM** USE
DILUTE BEFORE
INTRAVENOUS USE
ELKINS-SINN, INC.
CHERRY HILL, NJ 08003

FIGURE 4–103 • Gentamicin sulfate (Courtesy of Elkins-Sinn, Inc.).

DIRECTIONS: For intermittent IV infusion to adults, dilute drug in 50–200 mL isotonic saline or D-5-W and infuse over ½–2 h. Do not mix with other drugs.

8. ORDERED: Diphenhydramine 40 mg IV stat over 15 min and KVO with D-5-W
   AVAILABLE: Diphenhydramine hydrochloride 50 mg/mL in 1 mL Dosette vials; 50, 100, 250, and 1000 mL D-5-W; and imed 927 Volumetric Infusion Pump

Problem   **Answer**

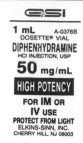

FIGURE 4–104 • Diphenhydramine hydrochloride (Courtesy of Elkins-Sinn, Inc.).

DIRECTIONS: Give IM or slow IV. Adult dose is 10–50 mg deep IM or IV up to 100 mg with maximum daily dosage of 400 mg.

9. ORDERED: Epinephrine IV push stat according to emergency room guidelines for 55 lb child and KVO with D-5-W

   AVAILABLE: Epinephrine 1:10,000 in 10 mL Abboject syringe; 50 mL bag of D-5-W; and imed 965 Microvolumetric Infusion Pump

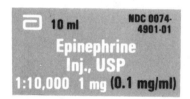

FIGURE 4–105 • Epinephrine (Courtesy of Abbott Laboratories).

DIRECTIONS: Emergency room standing orders guidelines are ''to give 0.01 mg/kg or 0.01 mL/kg of 1:10,000 epinephrine IV push into lowest portal.''

10. ORDERED: Atropine IV push stat according to pediatric intensive care unit standing emergency orders to a 44 lb child

Problem	Answer

AVAILABLE: Atropine sulfate 1 mg in 10 mL Abboject syringe and PCA PUMP infusing D-5-W at 50 mL/h

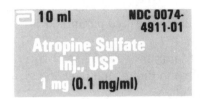

ⓐ **10 ml** **NDC 0074-4911-01**

Atropine Sulfate Inj., USP

1 mg (0.1 mg/ml)

FIGURE 4–106 • Atropine sulfate (Courtesy of Abbott Laboratories).

DIRECTIONS: Pediatric: intensive care unit standing emergency orders are ''to give 0.01 mg/kg IV push into lowest portal.''

SYRINGE INFUSERS

Syringe pumps are the third general type of machine for giving fluids intravenously. These machines move the plunger of the syringe very slowly and at the preset rate.

Syringe pumps are used when medications are to be given slowly over an extended period of time and when the volume of the drug solution is fairly small. When no other continuous IV fluids are being given, the drugs can be given by syringe infuser through a heparin lock. Otherwise, they can be given from the syringe infuser into various portals on the primary, secondary, burette, or volume delivery pump tubing, but preferably nearest the venipuncture site for reasons to be explained later (pp. 174–175). Depending on many factors, the flow of other fluids may or may not be interrupted while the syringe pump is operating.

Agency policies may call for use of additional medication and fluid to prime the tubing from the syringe. The amount will depend on the length and diameter of the tubing. Some tubing requires about 9 mL of fluid for priming. Microbore tubing is available for some syringe pumps.

Three of the available syringe infusers and their major capabilities follow:

- Harvard 2620 Syringe Infusion Pump (Harvard):
  - can use 50 mL B-D Plastipak or 60 mL Monoject plastic syringes
  - can be set to run at mL/h for up to 24 hours
- B-D 360 Infuser Syringe Pump System (Becton-Dickinson):
  - accommodates all 3 to 60 mL syringes
  - can run 10 to 60 minutes at 2.5-minute increments
- Auto Syringe (Baxter-Travenol):
  - will accommodate syringes from tuberculin to 60 mL size
  - can be set to run at mL/h for up to 24 hours

Some volume delivery pumps, such as some imeds, can be converted to syringe pumps. BARD's PCA pump will accommodate the B-D Plastipak or Sherwood Mono-ject plastic syringes.

Example Problems

Problem 1: ORDERED: Amikin 40 mg IV q12h by syringe pump and D-5-0.2 NS to run at 15 mL/h

AVAILABLE: Amikacin sulfate (Amikin) 100 mg in 2 mL vial; imed 965 Microvolumetric Infusion Pump; and B-D 360 syringe pump

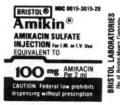

FIGURE 4–107 • Amikacin sulfate (Courtesy of Bristol Laboratories).

DIRECTIONS: Add 0.5 g to 100–200 mL of IV fluid. For children, use enough diluent to give over 30–60 min. For infants, use enough diluent to give over 1–2 h.

Solution:

$$100 \text{ mg} : 2 \text{ mL} = 40 \text{ mg} : x \text{ mL}$$
$$100x = 80$$
$$x = {}^{80}\!/_{100}$$
$$x = 0.8 \text{ mL of drug}$$

The practitioner decides to give the drug over a 2 h period.

$$15 \text{ mL} : 1 \text{ h} = x \text{ mL} : 2 \text{ h}$$
$$1x = 30 \text{ mL}$$

Answer: Put 0.8 mL of Amikin in a 50 mL syringe, fill to 30 mL, select the appropriate injection site, and set syringe pump to run at 15 mL/h.

Problem 2: ORDERED: Aminophyllin 40 mg/h by continuous IV in D-5-W and with a Harvard syringe infuser

AVAILABLE: Aminophylline (Aminophyllin) 500 mg/20 mL ampule

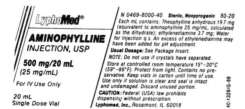

FIGURE 4–108 • Aminophylline (Courtesy of Lypho-Med, Inc.).

DIRECTIONS: Give very slowly IV by syringe or add to IV solution. Do not exceed 25 mg/min.

Solution:

$$40 \text{ mg}:1 \text{ h} = 500 \text{ mg}:x \text{ h}$$
$$40x = 500$$
$$x = {}^{500}\!/_{40}$$
$$x = 12.5 \text{ h}$$

Withdraw 20 mL of drug into a 60 mL Harvard syringe infuser; add 30 mL of D-5-W to drug in the syringe, leaving space in the syringe to mix the drug with the D-5-W; and calculate the rate at which the infuser is to be set.

$$500 \text{ mg}:50 \text{ mL} = 40 \text{ mg}:x \text{ mL}$$
$$500x = 2000$$
$$x = {}^{2000}\!/_{500}$$
$$x = 4 \text{ mL}$$

Answer: Adjust the infuser to deliver 4 mL/h. The drug solution will run 12.5 h. At the end of the 12 h, repeat the process. Or 40 mL of drug and 10 mL of IV solution could be set to run at 2 mL/h for 25 hours.

Problem 3: ORDERED: Regular human insulin 0.5 U/h by continuous 24 h IV via heparin lock

AVAILABLE: Regular human insulin (Novolin R insulin) 100 U, an Auto Syringe, and 60 mL syringe

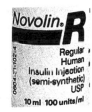

FIGURE 4–109 • Regular human insulin (Courtesy of Squibb-Nova, Inc.).

DIRECTIONS: No special directions are given.

Solution:

$$0.5 \text{ U}:1 \text{ h} = x \text{ U}:25 \text{ h}$$
$$x = 12.5 \text{ U}$$

If enough insulin to run 25 h is used, the syringe will not be completely empty at the end of 24 h, reducing the chances of blood clotting in the heparin lock.

Answer: Withdraw 12.5 U of regular human insulin, add to a 50 mL bag of appropriate IV fluid, mix, and withdraw all of IV fluid and insulin into a 60 mL syringe. Adjust Auto Syringe to run at 2 mL/h (50 mL:25 h = x mL:1 h).

Practice Problems

Answers can be found in Appendix C, p. 259.

Problem	**Answer**
1. ORDERED: Regular human insulin 1 U/h by continuous IV by heparin lock for 24 h administration	

Problem	**Answer**

AVAILABLE: Regular human
   insulin 100 U/mL, a Harvard
   syringe pump, and 60 mL
   Monoject plastic syringes

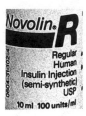

FIGURE 4–110 • Regular human insulin (Courtesy of Squibb-Nova, Inc.).

DIRECTIONS: No special directions
   given.

2. ORDERED: Heparin 800 U/h by
      continuous IV
   AVAILABLE: Heparin 1 mL vials
      10,000 U/mL and an Auto
      Syringe infuser

NDC 0009-0317-08   25—1 ml Vials

Heparin Sodium Injection, USP
Sterile Solution
10,000 Units per ml
from beef lung
For subcutaneous or intravenous use
Caution: Federal law prohibits dispensing without prescription.

FIGURE 4–111 • Heparin sodium (Courtesy of The Upjohn Company).

DIRECTIONS: Give IV undiluted or
   in IV solution.

3. ORDERED: Dobutamine 250
      mcg/min by continuous IV until
      condition stabilizes
   AVAILABLE: Dobutamine
      hydrochloride (Dobutrex)
      250 mg/20 mL vials, an Auto
      Syringe infuser, and 50 mL
      syringes

Problem	**Answer**

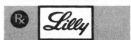

NDC 0002-7175-01
20 mL   VIAL No. 7175

DOBUTREX® SOLUTION
DOBUTAMINE HYDROCHLORIDE INJECTION
Equiv. to
250 mg
Dobutamine per 20 mL
**For I.V. Use Only
Must be diluted
prior to use**
CAUTION—Federal (U.S.A.) law prohibits dispensing without prescription.

FIGURE 4–112 • Dobutamine hydrochloride (Courtesy of Eli Lilly Industries, Inc.).

DIRECTIONS: Add 10 mL of diluent and, if not dissolved, add another 10 mL of diluent. Further dilute to at least 50 mL and use within 24 h.

4. ORDERED: Mefoxin 500 mg IV q6h with IV of D-5-W at 40 mL/h
AVAILABLE: Cefoxitin sodium (Mefoxin) 1 g vials, a B-D 360 syringe pump, and 30 and 60 mL syringes

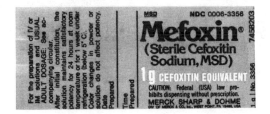

FIGURE 4–113 • Cefoxitin sodium (Courtesy of Merck Sharp & Dohme).

DIRECTIONS: Reconstitute 1 g with at least 10 mL of sterile water or 50–100 mL of appropriate IV solution. Hospital practice calls for infusion into Y portal nearest the venipuncture.

Problem	**Answer**

5. ORDERED: Dopamine 7
mcg/kg/min IV to infant
weighing 6 kg, and IV of
D-5-W at KVO
AVAILABLE: Dopamine 200 mg in
5 mL ampule, 50 mL bags of
D-5-W, and Auto Syringe

5 mL DOSETTE® AMPUL   A-1416d
6505-00-127-2923
DOPAMINE
HCl INJECTION, USP
200 mg/5 mL
(40 mg/mL equivalent to 32.3 mg base)
FOR **IV** INFUSION ONLY
POTENT DRUG: MUST DILUTE BEFORE USING
ESi ELKINS-SINN, INC.
CHERRY HILL, NJ 08003

FIGURE   4–114 • Dopamine   hydrochloride
(Courtesy of Elkins-Sinn, Inc.).

DIRECTIONS: No special directions
given.

6. ORDERED: Heparin 10,000 U IV
stat, then 5000 U q4h over 30
min in 50 mL of 0.9% sodium
chloride via heparin lock
AVAILABLE: Heparin sodium 5000
U/mL in 10 mL vial, 50 mL
bags of 0.9% NaCl, and
Harvard syringe infuser

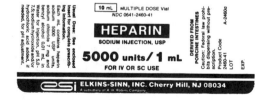

FIGURE 4–115 • Heparin sodium (Courtesy of
Elkins-Sinn, Inc.).

DIRECTIONS: For intermittent IV
infusion, give undiluted or in
50–100 mL of 0.9% NaCl.

7. ORDERED: Gentamicin 75 mg IV
q8h over 2 h via heparin lock
AVAILABLE: Gentamicin sulfate
80 mg/2 mL, 50 mL bags of
isotonic saline, and B-D 360
syringe pump

Problem   **Answer**

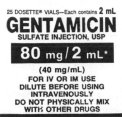

FIGURE 4–116 • Gentamicin sulfate (Courtesy of Elkins-Sinn, Inc.).

DIRECTIONS: For intermittent IV infusion in adults, dilute drug in 50–200 mL isotonic saline and infuse over ½–2 h. Do not mix with other drugs.

8. ORDERED: Pentam 200 mg IV qd for 14 days via heparin lock
AVAILABLE: Pentamidine isethionate (Pentam) 300 mg vials, 50 mL bags of D-5-W, and Harvard syringe infuser

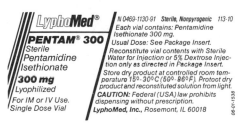

FIGURE 4–117 • Pentamidine isethionate (Courtesy of LyphoMed, Inc.).

DIRECTIONS: Dissolve contents of vial in 3–5 mL of sterile water. Add ordered amount of drug to 50–250 mL of D-5-W and infuse over 60 min. Closely monitor blood pressure during and after administration, and have emergency resuscitation equipment available.

PART 18 • Special Considerations for Intravenous Therapy

PORTALS OF ADMINISTRATION

One needs to consider the concentration and the rate of flow of the drug for two major reasons. First, the drug needs to be given at a rate and at a concentration that will ensure the attainment of therapeutic blood serum levels. Second, many drugs are irritating to the veins and further dilution of the drug often reduces this irritation. Drug literature enclosed with the drug container provides concentration recommendations. Sometimes it is acceptable to give drugs at concentrations greater than those recommended in order to prevent fluid overload, but certain drugs should never be given at greater than recommended concentrations.

Several research studies involving the administration of IV drugs to infants and children have shown that therapeutic serum levels were not always being attained when drugs were added to the primary IV high in the system—for example, into fluid volume control chambers.

In general, researchers have concluded that the more the rate of flow and/or the volume of IV fluid containing the drug decreases, the closer the portal of injection of the drug solution into the IV system should be to the venipuncture site, in order to increase the amount of drug that is infused. Their reasons are as follows:

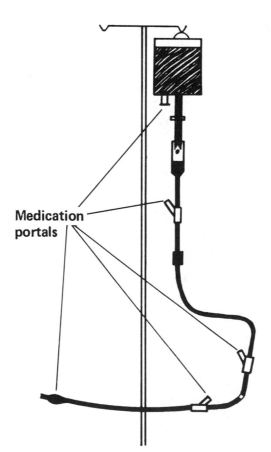

Medication portals

FIGURE 4–118 • Possible medication injection sites.

- Drugs have been found to adhere to filters and tubing throughout the system
- Drugs with a specific gravity lower than that of the primary IV solution tend to rise and remain in the IV tubing
- Drugs with a specific gravity higher than that of the primary solution tend to fall and remain in any low loop of tubing
- The more distal from the patient's vein that the drug is added to the system, the more drug that is discarded when the primary IV tubing is changed to fulfill infection control measures (the policy in most agencies calls for changing the IV fluid bags and administration sets at least every 24 hours)

For these reasons, the staff in some hospitals have protocols or policies to be used for selecting the drug injection site (Fig. 4–118 gives locations of possible injection sites).

STEPS IN SOLVING INTRAVENOUS DRUG PROBLEMS

The steps in IV medication problems are summarized here:

1. Amount of drug? Determined by the:
   - Physician's order
   - Practitioner who:
     - may have to reconstitute the drug

       and/or

     - usually has to convert g, mg, mcg, gr, U, or mEq ordered to number of mL to be given
2. Put drug in how many milliliters of IV fluid? This is affected by:
   - The type of administration which:
     - the physician may order

       or

     - the concentration of the drug solution that will be expressed as mcg, mg, g, U, or mEq/mL, which may be by physicians order or concentrations recommended in the drug literature
   - The practitioner's choice to do one of the following:
     - put the drug into total IV
     - put the drug into PB bags, the amount being limited to the capacity of the bags available unless some of the solution is withdrawn
     - put the drug into a volume control chamber and, possibly, add primary fluid
     - give the drug by IV push into heparin lock or IV tubing portals, the amount being limited by the size of the syringe, usually 20 or 30 mL maximum
     - give the drug by syringe pump into heparin lock or IV tubing portal, the amount being limited by the size of the syringes, usually 1 to 60 mL
3. Rate of administration? Practitioner may administer at the rate the:
   - Physician orders

     or

   - Literature recommends, eg:
     - give a certain amount of drug per minute or hour
     - administer the drug over or within a given period of time, such as in 20 minutes or 1 hour

- Practitioner judges to be reasonable in gtts/min, mL/min, or mL/h at:
  - the same rate as the primary IV is running

or

  - a different rate than the primary IV is running

CALCULATION OF FLUID NEEDS

Health practitioners need to be able to calculate fluid maintenance needs. One method that is used occasionally, especially with pediatric patients, is to use the guide of 1500 mL/m²/day.

Guide 1: 1500 mL/m²/day

A 30 lb child with a body surface area (BSA) of 0.6 m² would need 900 mL/day or 37.5 mL/h.

$$1500 \text{ mL} \times 0.6 \text{ m}^2 = 900 \text{ mL/day or } 37.5 \text{ mL/h}$$

Another guide many physicians consider to be more accurate and one that can be used for adults as well as children is as follows:

Guide 2: (1) 100 mL/kg for the first 10 kg
(2)   50 mL/kg for the next 10 kg
(3)   20 mL/kg for weight over 20 kg

A 220 lb (100 kg) man with no need for fluid restriction would need 3100 mL/day for maintenance or 129 mL/h.

1. 100 mL/kg for first 10 kg   = 1000 mL
2. 50 mL/kg for next 10 kg   = 500 mL
3. 20 mL/kg for weight over 20 kg = 1600 mL
                                     ─────────
                                     3100 mL

$$\begin{array}{r} 100 \text{ kg} \\ - 20 \text{ kg} \text{ (for first and second 10 kg)} \\ \hline 80 \text{ kg} \end{array}$$

$$20 \text{ mL} : 1 \text{ kg} = x \text{ mL} : 80 \text{ kg}$$
$$1x = 1600 \text{ mL}$$

$$3100 \text{ mL/day or } 129 \text{ mL/h for 24 h}$$

An 11 lb (5 kg) infant would need 500 mL/day or 21 mL/h or approximately 2 oz q3h if receiving oral fluids.

$$100 \text{ mL} : 1 \text{ kg} = x \text{ mL} : 5 \text{ kg}$$
$$x = 500 \text{ mL/day or } 20.8 \text{ mL/h for 24 h}$$

Using Guide 1, this 11 lb (0.29 m²) infant would need 435 mL/h.

$$1500 \text{ mL} \times 0.29 \text{ m}^2 = 435 \text{ mL/day or } 18.125 \text{ mL/h for 24 h}$$

Neonates (up to 1 month of age) require proportionately more fluid for their weight. Also, as one example, patients with cerebral edema may be given only ⅔ or ¾ of their calculated maintenance needs.

Example Problems

Problem 1: What are the normal daily fluid needs of a 52 lb (0.9 m^2) child using Guide 1?

Solution: $1500 \text{ mL} \times 0.9 \text{ m}^2 = 1350 \text{ mL/day}$

Answer: The child's fluid needs are 1350 mL/day.

Problem 2: What are the daily fluid needs of a normal 110 lb (50 kg) woman using Guide 2?

Solution:

    1. 100 mL/kg for first 10 kg   = 1000 mL
    2. 50 mL/kg for next 10 kg   =   500 mL
    3. 20 mL/kg for weight over 20 kg =   600 mL
                                            2100 mL/day

Answer: The woman's fluid needs are 2100 mL/day.

Problem 3: What are the normal q3h fluid needs of an 8 lb, 8 oz newborn (BSA $= 0.245 \text{ m}^2$), using Guide 1?

Solution: $1500 \text{ mL} \times 0.245 = 367.5 \text{ mL/day}$

There are eight 3 h periods in 24 h; therefore,

$$367.5 \text{ mL/day} \div 8 = 45.9 \text{ mL q3h}$$

Answer: The newborn's fluid needs are 46 mL every 3 hours.

Problem 4: What are the normal q3h fluid needs of an 8 lb, 8 oz newborn, using Guide 2?

Solution: 100 mL/kg for first 10 kg = 100 mL $\times$ 4 kg = 400 mL/day
                                400 mL/day $\div$ 8 = 50 mL q3h

Answer: The newborn's fluid needs are 50 mL every 3 hours.

Practice Problems

Answers can be found in Appendix C, pp. 259–260.

Problem	Answer
1. What are the daily fluid needs of a normal 165 lb man, using Guide 2?	

Problem	**Answer**

2. What are the q3h fluid needs of a 6-lb (0.2 m^2) normal infant, using Guide 1?

3. What are the q4h fluid needs of a normal infant weighing 11 lb, using Guide 2?

4. What are the q4h fluid needs of a normal infant weighing 11 lb (0.29 m^2), using Guide 1?

5. What are the daily fluid needs of a 100 lb woman, using Guide 2?

Problem	Answer

6. What are the q4h fluid needs of a 2-year-old child (0.6 m²), using Guide 1?

7. What are the daily fluid needs of a 10-year-old boy (1.2 m²) using Guide 1?

8. What are the hourly fluid needs of a 22 lb child receiving IV fluids and nothing by mouth, using Guide 2?

CALCULATION OF CALORIES IN INTRAVENOUS FLUIDS

An instance in which caloric intake may need to be calculated is when the patient is receiving intravenous (IV) fluids only by peripheral veins. Usually the maximum amount of fluid given IV in a 24-hour period to an adult is approximately 3000 mL. Often this is a 5% dextrose solution. A 5% dextrose solution contains 5 g of dextrose in every 100 mL of solution. Using Formula B one can calculate the total calories that a patient will receive in 24 hours if he or she receives 3000 mL of D-5-W. Although there are 4 calories per g of carbohydrates, there are actually only 3.4 calories per g of dextrose.

$$5 \text{ g}:100 \text{ mL} = x \text{ g}:3000 \text{ mL}$$
$$100x = 15,000$$
$$x = {}^{15,000}\!/_{100}$$
$$x = 150 \text{ g}$$

$$
\begin{array}{r}
\times 3.4 \text{ (calories/g)} \\
\hline
600 \\
450 \quad\;\; \\
\hline
510.0 \text{ calories}
\end{array}
$$

In a 24-hour period, the patient would receive only 510 calories; these are carbohydrate calories only.

Example Problems

Problem 1: How many calories are there in 1500 mL of D-5-W and 500 mL of 0.45% sodium chloride given over 24 h?

Solution:
$$5 \text{ g}:100 \text{ mL} = x \text{ g}:1500 \text{ mL}$$
$$100x = 7500$$
$$x = {7500}/{100}$$
$$x = 75 \text{ g dextrose}$$
$$\begin{array}{r} \times 3.4 \text{ calories/g} \\ \hline 300 \\ 225 \\ \hline 255.0 \text{ calories} \end{array}$$

Answer: There are a total of 255 calories in the 1500 mL of D-5-W and no calories in the 500 mL of 0.45% sodium chloride.

Problem 2: How many calories are there in 500 mL of D-5-W given in 24 h to an 11 lb infant?

Solution:
$$5 \text{ g}:100 \text{ mL} = x \text{ g}:500 \text{ mL}$$
$$100x = 2500$$
$$x = {2500}/{100}$$
$$x = 25 \text{ g dextrose}$$
$$\begin{array}{r} \times 3.4 \text{ calories/g} \\ \hline 100 \\ 75 \\ \hline 85.0 \text{ calories} \end{array}$$

Answer: There are 85 calories in the 500 mL of D-5-W solution.

Even high nutritional needs can be met with total parenteral nutrition (TPN). These hypertonic solutions of essential amino acids, dextrose, fatty acids, electrolytes, minerals, and vitamins used to be administered into the superior vena cava via the sub-clavian vein. Currently, TPN solutions are given into almost any vein, including peripheral veins. These solutions are ordered by the physician and prepared in the pharmacy. Supplements of essential fatty acids or lipids usually are given daily over 12 to 18 hours, or as part of the TPN. When high concentrations of amino acids or proteins (4 calories/g), fatty acids (11 calories/g), and dextrose (3.4 calories/g) are given, even high caloric needs can be met.

Problem 3: How many calories are there in 3 liters/day of TPN of 12% dextrose and 3.5% amino acids?

Solution:
$$12 \text{ g}:100 \text{ mL} = x \text{ g}:3000 \text{ mL}$$
$$100 \text{ x} = 36,000$$
$$x = {36,000}/{100}$$

$$x = 360 \text{ g dextrose}$$
$$\underline{\times 3.4 \text{ calories/g}}$$
$$1440$$
$$\underline{1080}$$
$$1224.0 \text{ calories from dextrose}$$

$$3.5 \text{ g}:100 \text{ mL} = x \text{ g}:3000 \text{ mL}$$
$$100 \text{ x} = 10{,}500$$
$$x = {}^{10{,}500}\!/_{100}$$
$$x = 105 \text{ g amino acids}$$
$$\underline{\times 4 \text{ calories/g}}$$
$$420 \text{ calories from amino acids}$$

Answer: Total calories equal 1644 (1224 from the dextrose and 420 from the amino acids).

Problem 4: How many calories are there in each 500 mL of 10% fat emulsion (11 calories/g) supplement given daily?

Solution:

$$10 \text{ g}:100 \text{ mL} = x \text{ g}:500 \text{ mL}$$
$$100 \text{ x} = 5000$$
$$x = {}^{5000}\!/_{100}$$
$$x = 50 \text{ g fat}$$
$$\underline{\times 11 \text{ calories/g}}$$
$$50$$
$$\underline{50}$$
$$550 \text{ calories}$$

Answer: Each 500 mL of 10% fat emulsion contains 550 calories.

Practice Problems:

Answers can be found in Appendix C, p. 260.

Problem	Answer
1. How many calories are there in 2000 mL of D-5-W?	
2. How many calories are there in 500 mL of D-10-W?	

Problem	**Answer**

3.   How many calories are there in 200 mL of TPN of 25% dextrose and 3.5% amino acids plus 500 mL of 10% fat emulsion?

4.   How many calories are there in 500 mL of 20% fat emulsion?

5.   How many calories are there in 1000 mL of 3.5% amino acids, 10% lipids, and 12% dextrose?

6.   How many calories are there in 500 mL of 3.5% amino acids, 10% fatty acids, and 10% dextrose?

Problem	**Answer**

7. How many calories are there in
   1500 mL of 3.5% amino acids?

8. How many calories are there in
   500 mL of 20% lipids, 3.5%
   amino acids, and 12%
   dextrose?

Pediatric and Geriatric Dosages

OBJECTIVES

At the end of this chapter, the student should be able to:
- Understand some of the many factors affecting drug absorption, distribution, metabolism, and elimination in infants and young children
- Calculate correct pediatric dosages
- Understand some of the many factors affecting drug absorption, distribution, metabolism, and elimination in older patients

PART 19 • Determination of Safe Pediatric Dosages

PHYSIOLOGIC DIFFERENCES

The physiologic processes of infants and young children are not fully matured. Consequently, the absorption, distribution, metabolism, and elimination of drugs is different in infants and children, sometimes enhanced, delayed, or decreased.

Usually drug absorption is delayed in infants and small children due to several immature processes; however, the nature of the drug itself also must be considered. For example, due to lower gastric acidity, the pH of the drug may delay or may accelerate absorption. The topical absorption of drugs by the young is enhanced. Intramuscular absorption varies with muscle mass.

Several physiologic differences affect the distribution of drugs in pediatric patients. These differences usually result in wider, faster distribution of the drug, thus threatening toxicity. However, the distribution of some drugs is delayed. An infant's decreased sensitivity to certain drugs requires higher doses per unit body weight than in adults.

The metabolism of most drugs is lower in infants, but some drugs increase the rate and extent of metabolism of the drug. The elimination of drugs by the kidneys is decreased until 1 year of age.

185

Normally, all physiologic processes are matured by age 12. Sometimes the pathologic condition, such as meningitis, warrants the administration of massive amounts of drugs to infants and children.

Because so many variables may affect the pediatric patients' response to drug therapy, it behooves the practitioner to assess for signs of toxicity or inadequate responses of each child to the prescribed drug regimen.

In past years, Young's, Fried's, and Clark's rules were commonly used for determining dosages for infants and children. Rarely used today, these rules are included in Appendix B for the convenience of some practitioners, but example problems involving their use are not included here.

DOSAGE BASED ON BODY WEIGHT

Most often pharmaceutical companies state the recommended dosages as the amount of drug per kilogram of body weight for 24 hours in divided doses. The dosages for pediatric patients are drug specific, that is, one drug may have a specific dosage recommendation different from that of any other drug. Some disease conditions are treated with unusually high dosages of medications. Also, the recommended dosage for a specific drug often varies with the age and condition of the infant or child. For example:

- To infants 0 to 1 week old, give 75 mg/kg q12h; to infants 1 week to 1 month old, give 75 mg/kg q8h; and to children 1 month to 12 years old, give 50 mg/kg q4h
- The maintenance dose for children is 0.7 mg/kg/day divided into three doses
- Give children and infants 50 to 100 mg/kg/day divided q4 to 8h; with mild renal impairment give 0.75 to 1.5 g q6h
- For children with meningitis, give 200 mg/kg/day in divided doses

In summary, pediatric dosages may be:

- Different for each age group
- Drug specific
- Higher for meningitis and other serious infections and/or disease conditions

Remember that 1 kg = 2.2 lb. Therefore, an adult weighing 220 lb weighs 100 kg.

$$1 \text{ kg} : 2.2 \text{ lb} = x \text{ kg} : 220 \text{ lb}$$
$$2.2x = 220$$
$$x = {}^{220}\!/_{2.2}$$
$$x = 100 \text{ kg}$$

An infant weighing 11 lb weighs 5 kg.

$$1 \text{ kg} : 2.2 \text{ lb} = x \text{ kg} : 11 \text{ lb}$$
$$2.2x = 11$$
$$x = {}^{11}\!/_{2.2}$$
$$x = 5 \text{ kg}$$

DOSAGE BASED ON BODY SURFACE AREA

Some physicians believe that the use of body surface area (BSA) is the most accurate method of estimating safe dosages for infants and children weighing less than 10 kg because the BSA is thought to be more closely related to infants' or children's metabolism than is their weight. However, the use of BSA for calculating dosages for infants weighing less than 10 kg will result in dosages higher than those based on kilograms of body weight, and these dosages would prove to be excessive doses.

Pharmaceutical companies may state a specific amount of recommended drug as so much drug:

- **Per m² of BSA**
- **Per kilogram of body weight**

NOMOGRAM

To determine the BSA in square meters (m^2), one uses a nomogram (Fig. 5–1). In practice, the calculation of BSA by nomogram is more often used to determine fluid replacement needs than to determine medication dosages. To use a nomogram, one:

- Plots the child's height on the far left vertical column
- Plots the child's weight on the far right vertical column
- Places a straightedge connecting the vertically plotted height and weight dots and draws a line between the two dots
- Determines the BSA in m^2 at the point at which the straightedge crosses the surface area (SA) scale

For example, if a child's weight is 24 lb and height 28 inches, the BSA would be $0.28 \ m^2$.

When the child is of normal height for weight, weight in pounds alone can be used to determine BSA, using the blocked area on the nomogram. If the child weighs 50 lb, then the BSA would be $0.88 \ m^2$. Simply plot the weight in pounds on the left column in the blocked area in the center of the nomogram and read the BSA from the numbers to the right of the line.

A formula for determining the amount of drug to be given if the amount of drug per m^2 is not given is shown here.

$$\frac{\text{BSA in } m^2 \times \text{adult dose}}{1.7} = \text{Infant's or child's dose}$$

The 1.7 in this formula represents the average adult BSA in square meters. When directions specify the amount of drug to be given per m^2 of BSA, this formula is not needed.

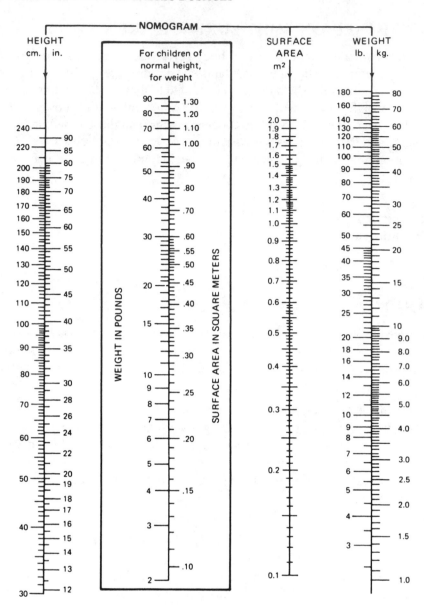

FIGURE 5–1 • The West nomogram for body surface area (BSA). (From Deglin, JH and Vallerand, AH: Davis Drug Guide for Nurses. F.A. Davis Co., Philadelphia, 1988, p 707).

Example Problems

Problem 1: ORDERED: Cleocin 60 mg IM q6h for a 2-month-old infant, height 22 inches and weight 6 kg

AVAILABLE: Clindamycin phosphate (Cleocin) 300 mg in 2 mL vials

NDC 0009-0870-21   25—2 ml Vials (single dose containers)
6505-01-185-3309

Cleocin Phosphate® 300 mg

Sterile Solution
clindamycin phosphate injection, USP
Equivalent to **300 mg** clindamycin
For intramuscular or intravenous use
Caution: Federal law prohibits dispensing without prescription.

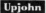

FIGURE 5–2 • Clindamycin phosphate (Courtesy of The Upjohn Company).

DIRECTIONS: For children older than 1 month of age, give 20–40 mg/kg/day in four equal doses.

Solution: 6 kg × 40 mg = 240 mg maximum per day

60 mg × 4 times a day = 240 mg ordered per day

The amount ordered falls within the guidelines of the directions.

150 mg : 2 mL = 60 mg : x mL

150x = 120

$x = {}^{120}\!/_{150}$

x = 0.8 mL

Answer: Give 0.8 mL of clindamycin phosphate 150 mg/mL IM every 6 hours.

Problem 2: ORDERED: Demerol 5 mg IM q4h prn for a 15-month-old baby of normal height for weight

AVAILABLE: Meperidine hydrochloride (Demerol) 25 mg/0.5 mL ampules (this drug is a narcotic).

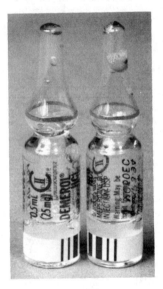

FIGURE 5–3 • Meperidine hydrochloride (From Winthrop Pharmaceuticals with permission).

DIRECTIONS: Adult dose is 50–100 mg q4h.

Solution: Use body surface area formula. (The nomogram scale for children of normal height for weight was used in determining the baby's BSA to be 0.57 m^2.)

$$\frac{0.57 \text{ m}^2 \times 100 \text{ mg}}{1.7} = x$$

$$x = \frac{57}{1.7}$$

x = 33.53 mg maximum per day

5 mg × 6 times a day = 30 mg ordered

The amount ordered is within safe limits.

25 mg : 0.5 mL = 5 mg : x mL

25x = 2.5

$x = {}^{2.5}\!/_{25}$

x = 0.1 mL

Answer: Using a tuberculin syringe, give 0.1 mL of meperidine hydrochloride 50 mg/mL IM every 4 hours as needed.

Problem 3: ORDERED: Morphine sulfate 4 mg IM q4h prn for pain for a 6-year-old child, weight 42 lb and height 45 inches

AVAILABLE: Morphine sulfate 8 mg (⅛ gr)/mL ampules. (This is a narcotic.)

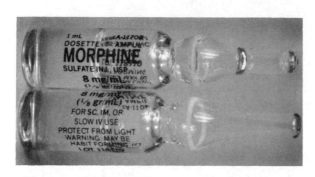

FIGURE 5–4 • Morphine sulfate (From Wyeth Laboratories, Inc., with permission).

DIRECTIONS: Usual adult dose is 15 mg; range is 8–20 mg.

Solution: Use body surface area formula. (The nomogram was used to determine that this child's BSA is 0.8 m².)

$$\frac{0.8 \text{ m}^2 \times 15 \text{ mg}}{1.7} = x$$

$$x = \frac{12}{1.7}$$

$$x = 7.06 \text{ mg maximum dose}$$

The ordered dose is reasonable since it is considerably less than the 7.06 mg determined to be within safe limits, but remember that this is a narcotic.

$$8 \text{ mg}:1 \text{ mL} = 4 \text{ mg}:x \text{ mL}$$
$$8x = 4$$
$$x = \tfrac{4}{8}$$
$$x = \tfrac{1}{2} \text{ or } 0.5 \text{ mL}$$

Answer: Using a tuberculin syringe, give 0.5 mL of morphine sulfate 8 mg/mL IM every 4 hours when needed for pain.

Problem 4: ORDERED: Claforan 200 mg IV q12h to a 1-week-old infant, weight 4000 g and length 18 inches

AVAILABLE: Cefotaxime sodium (Claforan) 95 mg/mL when 1 g vial is reconstituted as directed

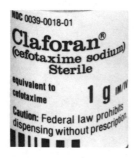

FIGURE 5–5 • Cefotaxime sodium (Courtesy of Hoescht-Roussel Pharmaceuticals, Inc.).

DIRECTIONS: Newborn to 1 week give 50 mg/kg q12h

Solution:

$$\text{Remember that } 1000 \text{ g} = 1 \text{ kg so } 4000 \text{ g} = 4 \text{ kg}$$
$$50 \text{ mg} : 1 \text{ kg} = x \text{ mg} : 4 \text{ kg}$$
$$x = 200 \text{ mg}$$

The amount ordered is equal to the recommended dose of 50 mg/kg q12h.

$$95 \text{ mg} : 1 \text{ mL} = 200 \text{ mg} : x \text{ mL}$$
$$95x = 200$$
$$x = {}^{200}\!/_{95}$$
$$x = 2.1 \text{ mL}$$

Answer: Give the infant 2.1 mL of cefotaxime sodium 95 mg/mL in an appropriate amount of IV solution every 12 hours.

Practice Problems

Answers to problems may be found in Appendix C, pp. 260–262.

Problem	Answer

1. ORDERED: Tigan 100 mg PO tid for an 8-year-old child, weight 50 lb, height 48 inches
   AVAILABLE: Trimethobenzamide hydrochloride (Tigan) 100 mg capsules

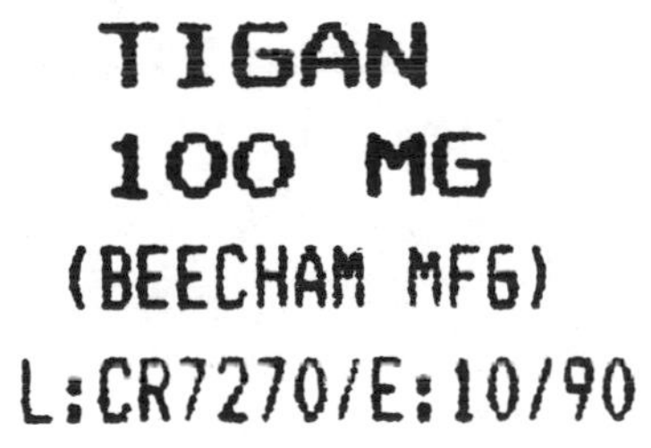

**TIGAN
100 MG
(BEECHAM MFG)
L:CR7270/E:10/90**

FIGURE 5–6 • Trimethobenzamide hydrochloride (From Beecham Laboratories with permission).

   DIRECTIONS: Adult dose is 250 mg capsules tid or qid.

2. ORDERED: Polycillin-N 100 mg IM q6h for a 1-year-old baby, weight 17.5 lb, normal height for weight
   AVAILABLE: Ampicillin sodium (Polycillin-N) 250 mg/mL when reconstituted as directed

Problem	**Answer**

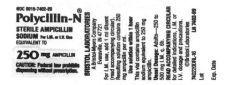

FIGURE 5–7 • Ampicillin sodium (Courtesy of Bristol Laboratories).

DIRECTIONS: For children, give 25–50 mg/kg/day in equally divided doses at 6 h intervals.

3. ORDERED: Amoxil oral suspension 75 mg q8h for 1-year-old child, weight 26 lb and normal height for weight
AVAILABLE: Amoxicillin (Amoxil) 125 mg/5 mL when reconstituted as directed

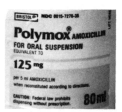

FIGURE 5–8 • Amoxicillin (From Bristol Laboratories with permission).

DIRECTIONS: Adult dose is 250 mg q8h and 20 mg/kg/day for children under 20 kg.

4. ORDERED: Ticar 250 mg IM q6h for a 5-year-old child, weight 44 lb, height 41 inches, with uncomplicated urinary infection
AVAILABLE: Ticarcillin disodium (Ticar) 1 g/2.6 mL when reconstituted as directed

Problem   **Answer**

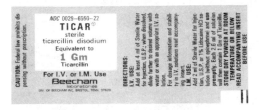

FIGURE 5–9 • Ticarcillin disodium (Courtesy of Beecham Laboratories).

DIRECTIONS: For uncomplicated urinary infection, give children weighing less than 40 kg 50–100 mg/kg/day in divided doses every 6–8h.

5. ORDERED: Cortone 12.5 mg PO qid, initial dose, for a 10-year-old, weight 64 lb, height 3 ft, 9 inches

AVAILABLE: Cortisone acetate (Cortone) 25 mg scored tablets

100 | No. 7063

TABLETS

CORTONE ® Acetate

(CORTISONE ACETATE, MSD)
25 mg

FIGURE 5–10 • Cortisone acetate (Courtesy of Merck Sharp & Dohme).

DIRECTIONS: Adult initial dose as much as 300 mg/day.

6. ORDERED: Clindamycin 100 mg IV q8h for 8-year-old, weight 55 lb, height 3 ft, 7 inches

AVAILABLE: Clindamycin phosphate (Cleocin) 150 mg/mL in 4 mL vials

Problem	**Answer**

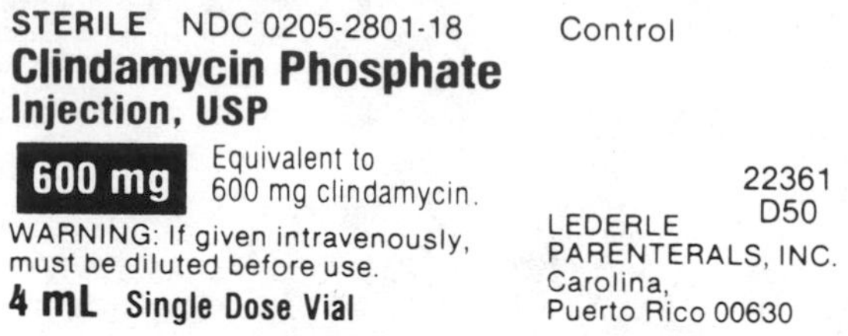

STERILE   NDC 0205-2801-18   Control
Clindamycin Phosphate
Injection, USP

600 mg   Equivalent to
            600 mg clindamycin.   22361
WARNING: If given intravenously,   LEDERLE   D50
must be diluted before use.   PARENTERALS, INC.
4 mL Single Dose Vial   Carolina,
                                    Puerto Rico 00630

FIGURE 5–11 • Clindamycin phosphate
(Courtesy of The Upjohn Company).

DIRECTIONS: For children, give
$350–450$ mg/m^2/day.

7. ORDERED: Robinul 0.05 mg IM
   preoperatively at 0700 h for a
   9-month-old infant, weight 8
   kg, height 70 cm
   AVAILABLE: Glycopyrrolate
   (Robinul) 0.2 mg/mL in 1 mL
   vial

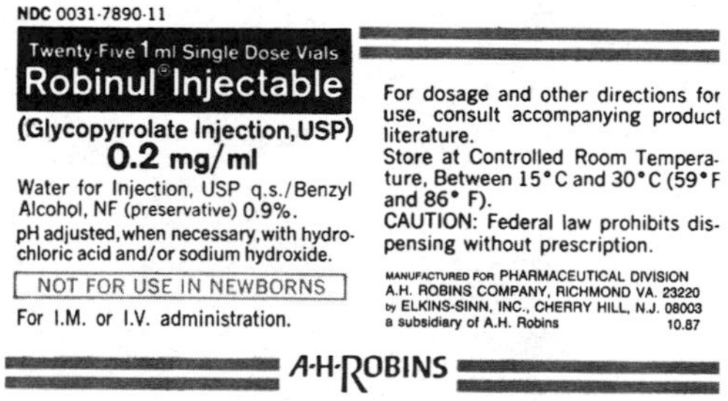

NDC 0031-7890-11

Twenty-Five **1** ml Single Dose Vials
Robinul® Injectable
(Glycopyrrolate Injection, USP)
0.2 mg/ml
Water for Injection, USP q.s./Benzyl
Alcohol, NF (preservative) 0.9%.
pH adjusted, when necessary, with hydro-
chloric acid and/or sodium hydroxide.

NOT FOR USE IN NEWBORNS

For I.M. or I.V. administration.

For dosage and other directions for
use, consult accompanying product
literature.
Store at Controlled Room Temperature, Between 15°C and 30°C (59°F
and 86°F).
CAUTION: Federal law prohibits dispensing without prescription.

MANUFACTURED FOR PHARMACEUTICAL DIVISION
A.H. ROBINS COMPANY, RICHMOND VA. 23220
by ELKINS-SINN, INC., CHERRY HILL, N.J. 08003
a subsidiary of A.H. Robins   10.87

A·H·ROBINS

FIGURE 5–12 • Glycopyrrolate (Courtesy of
A.H. Robins Co.).

DIRECTIONS: Recommended
   dose in children aged
   1 month–12 years is 0.002
   mg/lb IM, but children
   1 month–2 years old may
   require 0.004 mg/lb
   preoperatively.

8. ORDERED: Digoxin 50 mcg IV
   q12h today for a 4-year-old
   child, weight 20 kg, normal
   height for weight

Problem	**Answer**

AVAILABLE: Digoxin (Lanoxin) 100 mcg (0.1 mg) in 1 mL ampule

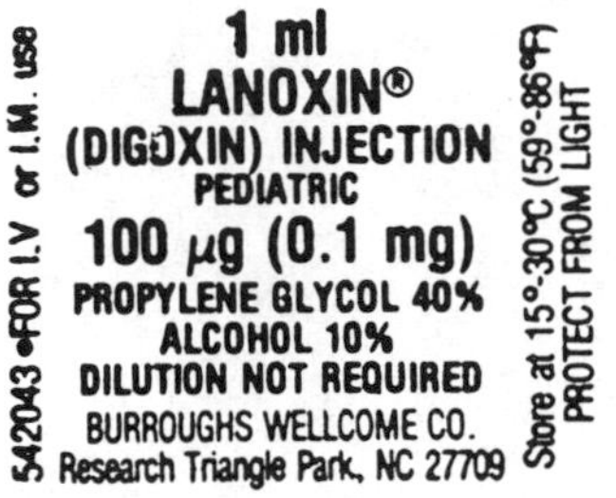

1 ml
LANOXIN®
(DIGOXIN) INJECTION
PEDIATRIC
100 μg (0.1 mg)
PROPYLENE GLYCOL 40%
ALCOHOL 10%
DILUTION NOT REQUIRED
BURROUGHS WELLCOME CO.
Research Triangle Park, NC 27709
542043 • FOR I.V. or I.M. use
Store at 15°-30°C (59°-86°F) PROTECT FROM LIGHT

FIGURE 5–13 • Digoxin (Courtesy of Burroughs Wellcome Co.).

DIRECTIONS: For children 2–5 years old digitalizing dose is 25–35 mcg/kg/day in divided doses.

9. ORDERED: Demerol 50 mg PO q4h prn for severe pain for a 7-year-old child, weight 40 lb, height 100 cm

AVAILABLE: Meperidine hydrochloride (Demerol) 50 mg tablets

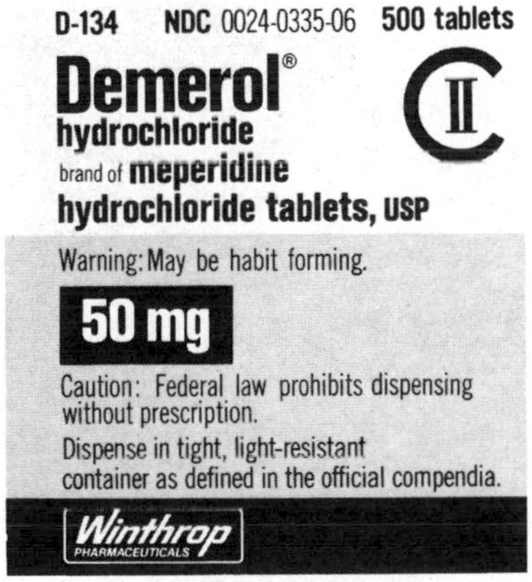

D-134   NDC 0024-0335-06   **500 tablets**

Demerol®
hydrochloride
brand of **meperidine**
hydrochloride tablets, USP

Warning: May be habit forming.

50 mg

Caution: Federal law prohibits dispensing without prescription.

Dispense in tight, light-resistant container as defined in the official compendia.

Winthrop
PHARMACEUTICALS

FIGURE 5–14 • Meperidine hydrochloride (Courtesy of Winthrop Pharmaceuticals).

DIRECTIONS: Give children 0.5– 0.8 mg/lb up to adult dose q3–4h. Usual adult dose is 50–150 mg q3–4h.

Problem	**Answer**

10. ORDERED: Amikin 40 mg IM q8h
    for a 2-year-old child, weight
    8.8 kg
    AVAILABLE: Amikacin sulfate
    (Amikin) 100 mg/2 mL

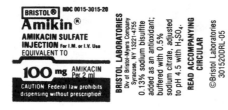

FIGURE 5–15 • Amikacin sulfate (Courtesy of Bristol Laboratories).

DIRECTIONS: For adults,
children, and infants give 7.5
mg/kg q12h or 5 mg/kg q8h.

11. ORDERED: Kantrex 20 mg IV q8h
    for a 1½-month-old infant,
    weight 4.25 kg
    AVAILABLE: Kanamycin sulfate
    (Kantrex) pediatric injection
    75 mg/2 mL when
    reconstituted as directed

FIGURE 5–16 • Kanamycin sulfate (Courtesy of Bristol Laboratories).

DIRECTIONS: Partial directions
are:

KG	MG/DAY
4.00	60.0
4.50	67.5

Problem	**Answer**

12. ORDERED: Chloramphenicol 500
    mg IV q6h for a 9-year-old
    child, weight 85 lb
    AVAILABLE: Chloramphenicol
    sodium succinate 1 g vial

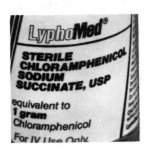

FIGURE 5–17 • Chloramphenicol sodium succinate (From Lypho Med, Inc. with permission).

DIRECTIONS: Give children 50
    mg/kg/day in four doses,
    depending on age, weight, and
    severity of infection. When
    reconstituted as directed,
    every mL will contain 100 mg.

13. ORDERED: Epinephrine 0.2 mg
    SC stat and q4h prn asthma for
    a 5-year-old child, weight 40 lb,
    normal height per weight
    AVAILABLE: Epinephrine 1:1000
    (1 mg/mL) in 1 mL Dosette
    ampules

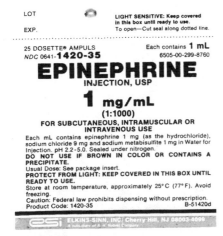

FIGURE 5–18 • Epinephrine (Courtesy of Elkins-Sinn, Inc.).

Problem	**Answer**

DIRECTIONS: For bronchial asthma in pediatric patients give 10 mcg/kg or 300 mcg/m^2 of BSA to a maximum of 500 mcg SC and repeat q4h if required.

14. ORDERED:Diphenhydramine 15 mg deep IM q6h today for a 2-year-old child weighing 22 lb, normal height per weight

AVAILABLE: Diphenhydramine 50 mg/mL in 1 mL Dosette vials

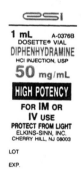

FIGURE 5–19 • Diphenhydramine (Courtesy of Elkins-Sinn, Inc.).

DIRECTIONS: Give children 5 mg/kg/24h or 150 mg/m^2/24h. Maximum daily dose is 300 mg divided into four doses.

15. ORDERED: Geopen 400 mg IV now, then 300 mg IV q6h for 3 days for 4000 g newborn

AVAILABLE: Carbenicillin disodium (Geopen) in a 2 g vial

Problem	**Answer**

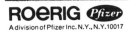

FIGURE 5–20 • Carbenicillin disodium (Courtesy of Roerig).

DIRECTIONS: For a 2 g vial:

DILUENT	1 G VOL
4.0 mL	2.5 mL
5.0 mL	3.0 mL
7.2 mL	4.0 mL

After reconstitution as directed, add to appropriate amount of IV fluid. For neonates weighing more than 2000 g, give 100 mg/kg as initial dose, 75 mg/kg q6h next 3 days, then 100 mg/kg q6h.

16. ORDERED: Gentamicin 10 mg IM q8h to 1-week-old infant weighing 9 lb
AVAILABLE: Gentamicin sulfate 20 mg/2 mL in Dosette vials

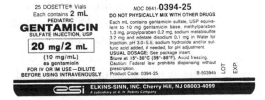

FIGURE 5–21 • Gentamicin sulfate (Courtesy of Elkins-Sinn, Inc.).

DIRECTIONS: Give infants and neonates 7.4 mg/kg/day in q8h doses.

Problem	**Answer**

17. ORDERED: Pfizerpen 200,000
U IM q6h to a newborn infant
AVAILABLE: Penicillin G
potassium 1,000,000 U in
20 mL vial

FIGURE 5–22 • Penicillin G potassium (Courtesy of Roerig).

DIRECTIONS: Give neonates
500,000 to 1 million U/day.
Dilutions for a 1,000,000 U vial:

DILUENT	U/mL
20.0 mL	50,000
10.0 mL	100,000
4.0 mL	250,000
1.8 mL	500,000

PART 20 • Considerations for Geriatric Drug Dosages

It is the immaturity of the physiologic processes that necessitates precautions in drug therapy for pediatric patients. For the elderly patient, it is the age changes in the physiologic functions that impose the need for special considerations of drug therapy. The increased incidence of long-standing disease processes results in multiple drug therapies that increase the chances of adverse drug reactions and interactions. Dosing schedules can be complicated and confusing, especially to those with mental and/or visual impairment. Socioeconomic factors affect the older person's ability to obtain the ever-increasingly expensive drugs. The aging process results in modifications in drug absorption, distribution, metabolism, and excretion.

Several causes of reduced gastrointestinal functioning result in reduced absorption of drugs. Drug interactions can inactivate or alter the action of some drugs. The use of many over-the-counter drugs can interfere with the actions of prescription drugs.

Despite delayed or reduced absorption, various physiologic changes increase or prolong the distribution of drugs, thus increasing the half-lives of drugs, sometimes leading to toxicity. Reduced blood flow decreases the metabolism of the drug by the liver, also prolonging the half-life of some drugs. Liver function, itself, also decreases during the aging process.

Reduced excretion of a drug is due to diminished renal function in the elderly. This is a major factor causing many changes in drug tolerance.

The elderly also experience increased sensitivity to certain drugs, especially drugs affecting the central nervous system. Like children, they may react to a drug in a way that is the opposite of the expected reaction.

All of these factors contribute to a small margin between a therapeutic dose and a toxic dose of a drug. Practitioners are challenged to monitor and manage the drug therapy of the elderly patient very closely.

Some institutions have set aside 1 day a week as a "drug holiday" on which no drugs are given. It is proposed that this time allows the patient a day for the slower physiologic processes to "catch up" with the drug administration. The efficacy of a drug holiday has not been proved by research studies.

CHAPTER

Comprehensive Review Problems

Answers to problems can be found in Appendix C, pp. 262–266.

Problem	Answer
1. 0.6 g = ? gr	
2. 50 mg = ? g	
3. 1½ gr = ? mg	

Problem	Answer

4. 50 mg = ? gr

5. ORDERED: Phenergan 15 mg IM
   q4h
   AVAILABLE: 1 mL ampules of
   promethazine hydrochloride
   (Phenergan) 25 mg/mL

6. ORDERED: 2000 mL D-5-W IV in
   24 h
   AVAILABLE: Abbott macrodrip
   administration set

7. ORDERED: Lente human insulin
   zinc suspension 50 U 1 h ac
   breakfast tomorrow
   AVAILABLE: Lente human
   insulin zinc suspension
   (Novolin L) 100 U and no
   insulin syringes

Problem	**Answer**

8. ORDERED: ASA 10 gr q3–4h prn
   for pain or fever over 102°F
   AVAILABLE: Acetylsalicylic acid
   (Aspirin) 300 mg tablets

9. ORDERED: Adrenalin 0.4 mg SC
   q3h prn for asthma
   AVAILABLE: 1 mL vial
   epinephrine (Adrenalin)
   1:1000

10. ORDERED: 25% alcohol cooling
    sponge prn (assume 1 qt is
    needed each time)
    AVAILABLE: 70% isopropyl
    alcohol

11. ORDERED: Vistaril 50 mg and
    Demerol 75 mg IM on call for
    surgery in AM
    AVAILABLE: Hydroxyzine
    hydrochloride (Vistaril) 50
    mg/mL in a 1 mL ampule and
    meperidine hydrochloride
    (Demerol) 100 mg/mL in 1
    mL ampule

Problem	**Answer**

12. ORDERED: Kantrex 25 mg IM
    q12h for an infant
    AVAILABLE: Kanamycin
    sulfate (Kantrex) solution
    75 mg/2 mL

13. ORDERED: Kaon Elixir 14 mEq
    tid
    AVAILABLE: A 4 oz bottle of
    potassium gluconate (Kaon)
    20 mEq/15 mL

14. ORDERED: Isotonic sodium
    chloride (NaCl) enema stat
    and prn (prepare 2 qt)
    AVAILABLE: Sodium chloride
    crystals

15. ORDERED: Aqueous buffered
    penicillin G 400,000 U IM
    q4h
    AVAILABLE: A 30 mL vial of
    penicillin G sodium 5,000,000
    U; to get 500,000 U/mL, add
    8 mL of diluent

Problem	**Answer**

16. ORDERED: Ferrous sulfate 5 gr
      PO tid
    AVAILABLE: Ferrous sulfate 300
      mg tablets

17. ORDERED: Elixir of phenobarbital
      30 mg PO tid
    AVAILABLE: Elixir of
      phenobarbital 20 mg/5 mL

18. ORDERED: Atropine sulfate gr
      1/200 IM stat
    AVAILABLE: Atropine sulfate 5
      mL (0.5 mg) in prefilled
      syringes

19. ORDERED: Regular human insulin
      15 U and NPH human insulin
      30 U ½ h ac breakfast
    AVAILABLE: Regular human
      insulin (Novolin R) 100 U/mL
      and NPH human insulin
      isophane suspension (Novolin
      N) 100 U/mL and 0.5 mL
      insulin syringe

Problem	Answer

20. ORDERED: Phenobarbital 30 mg
 PO qid
 AVAILABLE: Phenobarbital
 sodium tablets ¼ gr

21. ORDERED: Solu-Medrol 2 mg IV
 q6h for a 2 kg premature
 infant
 AVAILABLE: Methylprednisolone
 sodium succinate (Solu-
 Medrol) that when
 reconstituted contains 40 mg
 in 1 mL; and an imed 965
 Microvolumetric Infusion
 Pump set at 2 mL/h; and an
 Auto-Syringe
 DIRECTIONS: Give over at least
 30 min. Hospital policy for
 flow rate of less than 10 mL/h
 is to use tubing portal nearest
 patient and a syringe pump.

22. ORDERED: Phenobarbital 5 mg
 PO stat for a 1-year-old infant
 AVAILABLE: Phenobarbital
 sodium tablets 15 mg

Problem	**Answer**

23. ORDERED: Ampicillin 100 mg IV q6h and D-5-0.2 NS at 24 mL/h for a 1-year-old child

    AVAILABLE: Ampicillin sodium 125 mg vial, imed 960 Volumetric Infusion Pump with microdrop burette chamber and IV extension tubing

    DIRECTIONS: Add 1 mL to 125 mg vial to get 125 mg/mL. For direct IV add 5 mL diluent to 125 mg vial and give over 3–5 min. Hospital policy for 20–30 mL/h flow rate is to give by syringe into the portal on primary tubing nearest to the venipuncture site at 1 mL/min and to use a syringe pump for more than 5 mL of drug solution.

24. ORDERED: Ceclor 75 mg PO q8h for a 1-year-old child, weight 24 lb, height 30 inches (is this dose correct?)

    AVAILABLE: Cefaclor (Ceclor) oral suspension 125 mg/5 mL when mixed as directed in 75 mL bottle

    DIRECTIONS: Adult dose is 250 mg q8h. Child dose is 20 mg/kg/day divided into q8h doses.

Problem	**Answer**

25. ORDERED: Vistaril 20 mg IM stat for a 5-year-old child, weight 41 lb (is this dose correct?)

   AVAILABLE: Hydroxyzine hydrochloride (Vistaril) 25 mg/1 mL in 10 mL multidose vial

   DIRECTIONS: Child single dose is 0.5 mg/lb.

26. ORDERED: KVO with D-5-½ NS. Ampicillin 500 mg IV q6h at 0800, 1400, 2000, and 0200 h and Cleocin 400 mg IV q6h at 1200, 1800, 2400, and 0600 h, each within 1 h

   AVAILABLE: Ampicillin sodium, (Omnipen-N) 500 mg vial; Clindamycin phosphate (Cleocin) 150 mg/mL in 4 mL vial; drip chamber yielding 10 gtts/mL; and D-5-½ NS in 50 mL PB bags

   DIRECTIONS: Add 5 mL sterile water for injection to ampicillin 500 mg vial and use all of the reconstituted solution to yield 500 mg. Ampicillin is to be administered within 1 h after reconstitution. Clindamycin should be diluted to no more than 12 mg/mL and infusion rate should not exceed 30 mg/min.

Problem	**Answer**

27. ORDERED: Heparin 50 U IV push q6h and IV set at 1 mL/h for a 900 g premature infant

    AVAILABLE: AVI Micro 275 Volumetric Pump and heparin 100 U/mL in 1 mL Tubex syringes

    DIRECTIONS: May be given as available or may be diluted. Policy calls for the use of flashball, the tubing portal nearest the patient.

28. ORDERED: 1000 D-5-W to run 0800–1600 h today. At 1000 h, there is 600 mL left in the bag.

    AVAILABLE: Abbott macrodrip administration set

29. ORDERED: Lente human insulin zinc suspension 35 U and regular human insulin 10 U 20 min ac breakfast every AM

    AVAILABLE: Lente human insulin zinc suspension (Novolin L) 100 U/mL; regular human insulin (Novolin R) 100 U/mL; and no insulin syringe

Problem	Answer

30. ORDERED: Achromycin 250 mg q12h IV at a maximum of 100 mg/h and D-5-0.2 NS to run at 24 mL/h with imed 960 Volumetric Infusion Pump and microdrip burette for a 10-year-old child

AVAILABLE: Tetracycline hydrochloride (Achromycin) in 250 mg vial

DIRECTIONS: Add 5 mL of sterile water to get 250 mg of reconstituted drug. Further dilute in a minimum of 100 mL calcium-free IV solution (Ringer's and lactated Ringer's can be used). Rapid administration is to be avoided.

31. ORDERED: Tylenol 7½ gr prn headache

AVAILABLE: Acetaminophen 500 mg caplets (Extra-Strength Tylenol)

32. ORDERED: Morphine sulfate ¼ gr SC q3h prn pain

AVAILABLE: Morphine sulfate ⅛ gr/mL

Problem	**Answer**

33. ORDERED: 500 mL of a 2% boric
    acid solution for warm
    compress to lesion on left
    hand q4h
    AVAILABLE: 500 mL of a 5%
    boric acid solution and sterile
    water

34. ORDERED: 2 liters of 20% sodium
    bicarbonate solution for
    irrigation of both eyes stat
    AVAILABLE: Sodium bicarbonate
    powder and sterile water

35. 1:1000 = ? mg:1 mL

36. What are the hourly IV fluid needs
    of a 30 lb (0.6 m^2) child
    receiving nothing by mouth,
    using Guide 1?

Problem	**Answer**

37. ORDERED: Cleocin 75 mg IM q6h for a 6-month-old infant weighing 7.5 kg (Is the dose correct?)

AVAILABLE: Clindamycin phosphate (Cleocin) 150 mg/mL in 2 mL vials

DIRECTIONS: For children older than 1 month of age, give 20–40 mg/kg/day in four equal doses.

38. ORDERED: Tetracycline 0.5 g PO qid

AVAILABLE: Tetracycline oral suspension 250 mg/5 mL

39. ORDERED: 1000 mL D-5-W IV to run 1000–1800 h today. At 1400 h there are 250 mL left in the bag.

AVAILABLE: Baxter-Travenol macrodrip administration set

Problem	**Answer**

40. $1:1 = ?$ mg:1 mL

41. ORDERED: 1 qt of 0.45% normal
      saline PO over the next 4 h
      AVAILABLE: Table salt and tap
      water

42. ORDERED: 400 mL D-5-W IV in
      24 h
      AVAILABLE: Abbott microdrip
      administration set

43. What are the hourly IV needs of a
      90 lb (1.35 m^2) child receiving
      nothing by mouth, using
      Guide 1?

Problem	**Answer**

44. ORDERED: Claforan 175 mg IV q12h to a newborn infant weighing 3600 g (Is this dose correct?)

    AVAILABLE: Cefotaxime sodium (Claforan) 95 mg/mL when 1 g vial is reconstituted as directed.

    DIRECTIONS: To newborn to 1-week-old infant give 50 mg/kg q12h.

45. ORDERED: Donnatal 5 cc tid and hs

    AVAILABLE: 500 mL bottle of Elixir of Donnatal

46. ORDERED: 500 mL 0.45% sodium chloride IV in 2 h then 1000 mL D-5-W in 8 h

    AVAILABLE: Baxter-Travenol macrodrip administration set

47. 1:10,000 = ? mcg:1 mL

Problem	**Answer**

48. ORDERED: Mephoxin 750 mg IV q6h with IV of D-5-W at 50 mL/h

AVAILABLE: Cefoxitin sodium (Mefoxin) 1 g vials, a B-D 360 syringe pump, and 30 and 60 mL syringes

DIRECTIONS: Reconstitute 1 g with at least 10 mL of sterile water or 50–100 mL of appropriate IV solution. Hospital practice calls for infusion into Y portal nearest the venipuncture.

49. What are the daily fluid needs of a 200 lb man, using Guide 2?

50. ORDERED: Polycillin-N 100 mg IV q6h and D-5-W at 30 mL/h

AVAILABLE: Ampicillin sodium (Polycillin-N) 125 mg vial; IVAC 260 controller; a microdrip burette; and 500 mL bag of D-5-W

DIRECTIONS: Add 1.2 mL of diluent to get 125 mg/mL. Dilute to 2–30 mg/mL for IV use and give within 4 h.

Problem	**Answer**

51. 0.01 mg = ? mcg

52. ORDERED: Cortisone 0.005 g PO
      tid
    AVAILABLE: Cortisone acetate 10
      mg scored tablets

53. What are the q3h fluid needs of a
      newborn infant weighing 8 lb,
      using Guide 2?

54. ORDERED: Ampicillin 200 mg IM
      q4h
    AVAILABLE: Ampicillin in dry
      form: 125 mg, 250 mg, and 1
      g vials
    DIRECTIONS:

LABEL	**DILUENT**	**CONCENTRATION**
125 mg	1.0 mL	125 mg/mL
250 mg	0.9 mL	250 mg/mL
1 g	3.4 mL	250 mg/mL

Problem	**Answer**

55. ORDERED: Ampicillin 750 mg IM q8h

AVAILABLE: Same as in problem 54

DIRECTIONS: Same as in problem 54

56. ORDERED: Morphine sulfate 8 mg IM q4h prn for severe pain to a 5-year-old child, normal height for weight, weighing 40 lb (Is this dose correct?)

AVAILABLE: Morphine sulfate $\frac{1}{8}$ gr/mL ampules

DIRECTIONS: Usual adult dose is 15 mg; range is 8–20 mg.

57. $\frac{1}{60}$ gr = ? mg

Problem	**Answer**

58. ORDERED: Polycillin-N 250 mg
      IM q6h
    AVAILABLE: Polycillin-N in dry
      form in 1 g vial
    DIRECTIONS: Adding 3.4 mL of
      diluent to a 1 g vial yields 4
      mL of reconstituted solution.

59. ORDERED: 25 mL/h D-5-W IV
      over 24 h
    AVAILABLE: Baxter-Travenol
      microdrip administration set

60. How many calories are there in 500
      mL of 12% dextrose and 3.5%
      amino acids?

Problem	**Answer**

61. ORDERED: Pentam 150 mg IV qd and D-5-W at 25 mL/h

    AVAILABLE: Pentamidine isethionate (Pentam), 300 mg single-dose vial; IVAC 230 controller with microdrip burette; and 50, 100, and 250 mL PB bags of solution

    DIRECTIONS: Give adults and children 4 mg/kg once a day. Dissolve the contents of the vial in 3 mL of sterile water, dilute further in 50–250 mL of D-5-W, and infuse over 60 min.

62. ORDERED: Aminophyllin 100 mg IV PB in 1 h, then 35 mg/h for the next 12 h, and D-5-W at 65 mL/h

    AVAILABLE: Theophylline (Aminophylline) 80 mg/100 mL in 500 mL D-5-W IV bag; AVI 400 A Volumetric Infusion Pump; and 1000 mL bag of D-5-W

    DIRECTIONS: Do not give loading dose of drug faster than 25 mg/min. Theophylline is incompatible with many drugs.

Problem	**Answer**

63. 0.001 g = ? mg

64. How many calories are there in 1500 mL of 10% dextrose, 3.5% amino acids, and 10% lipids?

65. ORDERED: Nitropress 200 mcg/min IV for 5 min stat then titrate dose to BP plus KVO with D-5-W

    AVAILABLE: Sodium nitroprusside (Nitropress) 50 mg vial; LIFECARE 5000 PLUM infusion system with microdrip primary and secondary administration sets; and 250, 500, and 1000 mL bags of D-5-W

    DIRECTIONS: Dissolve drug in 2.3 mL of D-5-W; no other diluent should be used. Each 2 mL of reconstituted solution will contain 50 mg of the drug, which should be diluted further in 250–1000 mL of D-5-W. Promptly cover IV bag with drug and IV tubing with aluminum foil or other opaque material to protect from light.

Problem	**Answer**

66. ORDERED: Demerol 30 mg IM
q4h prn for a 50 lb child with
a BSA of 0.84 m^2 (Is this dose
correct?)
AVAILABLE: Meperidine
hydrochloride (Demerol) 50
mg/mL in 1 mL ampules.
DIRECTIONS: Adult dose is 50–
100 mg q4h

67. ORDERED: Dopamine 100
mcg/min initially in 250 mL
D-5-W
AVAILABLE: Dopamine 200 mg
in 5 mL ampules; 250 mL of
D-5-W; and imed 965
Microvolumetric Infusion
Pump
DIRECTIONS: Add 200 or 400 mg
to 250 or 500 mL,
respectively, of appropriate IV
fluid before infusing. Closely
observe vital signs and urinary
output.

68. ORDERED: Morphine ss gr IM
q4h prn pain
AVAILABLE: 10 mL vial of
morphine sulfate 30 mg/mL

Problem	**Answer**

69. ORDERED: Heparin 600 U/h by
continuous IV
AVAILABLE: Heparin 1 mL vial
10,000 U/mL and an Auto
Syringe Infuser
DIRECTIONS: Give IV undiluted
or in IV solution.

70. ORDERED: Hypaque 50 mg
intradermally
AVAILABLE: 50% Hypaque in 1
mL ampules

71. How many calories are there in
3000 mL of D-5-W?

Problem	**Answer**

72. ORDERED: 200 mL 5% glucose
     solution PO q4h for 24 h
     AVAILABLE: Sugar and distilled
     water

73. ORDERED: Regular human insulin
     0.75 U/h by continuous 24 h
     IV via heparin lock
     AVAILABLE: Regular human
     insulin 100 U/mL, a Harvard
     syringe pump, and 60 mL
     Monoject plastic syringes
     DIRECTIONS: No special
     directions given.

74. How many calories are there in 500
     mL D-10-W, 1000 mL of
     D-5-W, and 500 mL of 0.45%
     NaCl?

Problem	**Answer**

75. ORDERED: Lasix 10 mg IM at 0700 and 1900 h today only
    AVAILABLE: Furosemide (Lasix) 2 mL vial containing 20 mg

76. ORDERED: Staphcillin 300 mg IM q4h
    AVAILABLE: Methacillin sodium (Staphcillin) in dry form in a 6 g vial
    DIRECTIONS: For IM use, add 8.6 mL of diluent and each 2 mL will contain 1 g of staphcillin.

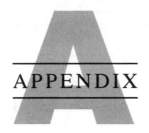

APPENDIX

Metric and Apothecaries' Equivalents

More detailed and/or exact apothecaries' and metric system equivalents are presented here for reference. There are very few areas that continue to use the apothecaries' system of measurement. Its use in dosage and solutions should be obsolete in a few years.

TABLE A–1 • Additional Approximate Metric/Apothecaries' Weight Equivalents		
Metric		**Apothecaries'**
	30 or 32 g	1 oz
	15 or 16 g	4 dr
	7.5 or 8 g	2 dr
	6 g	90 to 96 gr
	5 g	75 to 80 gr
	4 g	60 to 64 gr or 1 dr
	3 g	45 to 48 gr
	2 g	30 to 32 gr or ½ dr
	1.5 g	22½ to 24 gr
1000 mg	1 g	15 to 16 gr*
750 mg	0.75 g	11¼ to 12 gr
600 mg	0.6 g	9 to 9⅗ gr or 10 gr
500 mg	0.5 g	7½ to 8 gr
400 mg	0.4 g	6 to 6⅖ gr
300 mg	0.3 g	4½ to 4⅘ gr or 5 gr
250 mg	0.25 g	3¾ to 4 gr
200 mg	0.2 g	3 to 3⅕ gr
150 mg	0.15 g	2¼ to 2⅖ gr or 2½ gr
120 mg	0.12 g	1⅘ to 1⁹⁄₁₀ gr or 2 gr
100 mg	0.1 g	1½ to 1⅗ gr
75 mg	0.075 g	1⅛ to 1⅕ gr
60, 64, or 65 mg	0.06 to 0.065 g	1 gr
50 mg	0.05 g	¾ to ⅘ gr
40 mg	0.04 g	⅗ to ¹⁶⁄₂₅ gr *(continued)*

*Often when using both 15 and 16 gr = 1 g to determine these grain/gram equivalents, the answer is a fraction which is awkward to use. In such instances, a nearly equal, simplified fraction is listed also.

TABLE A–1 • Continued		
Metric		**Apothecaries'**
30 mg	0.03 g	$9/20$ to $12/25$ gr or $1/2$ gr
25 mg	0.025 g	$3/8$ to $2/5$ gr
20 mg	0.02 g	$3/10$ to $8/25$ gr or $1/3$ gr
15 mg	0.015 g	$9/40$ to $6/25$ gr or $1/4$ gr
12 mg	0.012 g	$9/50$ to $24/125$ gr or $1/5$ gr
10 mg	0.010 g	$3/20$ to $4/25$ gr or $1/6$ gr
8 mg	0.008 g	$·3/25$ to $16/125$ gr or $1/8$ gr
6 mg	0.006 g	$9/100$ to $12/125$ gr or $1/10$ gr
5 mg	0.005 g	$3/40$ to $2/25$ gr or $1/12$ gr
4 mg	0.004 g	$3/50$ to $8/125$ gr or $1/15$ to $1/16$ gr
3 mg	0.003 g	$9/200$ to $6/125$ gr or $1/20$ gr
2 mg	0.002 g	$3/100$ to $4/125$ gr or $1/30$ gr
1.5 mg	0.0015 g	$9/400$ to $3/125$ gr or $1/40$ gr
1.2 mg	0.0012 g	$9/500$ to $12/625$ gr or $1/50$ gr
1 mg	0.001 g	$3/200$ to $2/125$ gr or $1/60$, $1/64$, or $1/65$ gr
0.8 mg	0.0008 g	$3/250$ to $8/625$ gr or $1/80$ gr
0.6 mg	0.0006 g	$9/1000$ to $6/625$ gr or $1/100$ gr
0.5 mg	0.0005 g	$1/120$, $1/128$, or $1/130$ gr
0.4 mg	0.0004 g	$3/500$ to $4/625$ gr or $1/150$ to $1/160$ gr
0.3 mg	0.0003 g	$9/2000$ to $3/625$ gr or $1/200$ to $1/210$ gr
0.25 mg	0.00025 g	$3/800$ to $1/250$ gr
0.2 mg	0.0002 g	$3/1000$ to $2/625$ gr or $1/300$ to $1/320$ gr
0.15 mg	0.00015 g	$9/4000$ to $3/1250$ gr or $1/400$ gr
0.12 mg	0.00012 g	$9/5000$ to $6/3125$ gr or $1/500$ gr
0.1 mg	0.001 g	$3/2000$ to $1/625$ gr or $1/600$, $1/640$, or $1/650$ gr

TABLE A–2 • Exact Metric/Apothecaries' Equivalents	
12 Metric	**Apothecaries'**
31.1035 g	1 oz
1 g	15.432 gr
0.972 g	15 gr
0.648 g	10 gr
0.324 g	5 gr
0.0648 g	1 gr
1 mL	16.23 m

TABLE A–3 • **Approximate Apothecaries'/Metric Volume Equivalents**	
Apothecaries'	*Metric*
1 minim (m)	0.06–0.07 milliliter (mL)
4 m	0.25 mL
8 m	0.5 mL
15 or 16 m	1 mL or 1 cubic centimeter (cc)
1 fluid dram (fl dr) or 60 or 64 m	4 mL
1 fluid ounce (fl oz) or 8 fl dr	30 or 32 mL
1 pint (pt) or 16 fl oz	480 or 500 mL
1 quart (qt) or 32 fl oz	960 or 1000 mL or 1 liter
1 gallon (gal) or 128 fl oz	3840 or 4000 mL or 4 liters

TABLE A–4 • **Commonly Used Approximate Apothecaries'/Metric Weight Equivalents**	
Apothecaries'	*Metric*
1/60. 1/64, or 1/65 grain (gr)	1 milligram (mg) or 1000 micrograms (mcg)
1 gr	0.06, 0.064, or 0.065 gram (g)
1 gr	60, 64, or 65 mg
1 gr	60,000, 64,000, or 65,000 mcg
5 gr	0.3 or 0.33 g
10 gr	0.6 or 0.67 g
15 or 16 gr	1 g
1 dram (dr)	4 g
1 ounce (oz)	30 or 32 g
1 pound (lb) (avoirdupois)	450 g
1 lb	0.4536 kilogram (kg)
2.2 lb (imperial or avoirdupois—not apothecaries')	1 kg
2.6 lb (apothecaries'— which is not used by practitioners)	1 kg

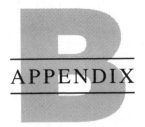

APPENDIX

Young's, Fried's and Clark's Rules

In past years, Young's, Fried's, and Clark's rules were commonly used for determining dosages for infants and children. These rules, rarely used today, are included for the convenience of some users. When used, the rules should serve as rough guides to determining approximate child dosages. It should be noted that Young's and Fried's rules do not allow for such important factors as the child's weight or body surface area.

YOUNG'S RULE (for children from 1 or 2 to 12 years)

$$\frac{\text{Age in years}}{\text{Age plus 12}} \times \text{Adult dose} = \text{Child's dose}$$

FRIED'S RULE (for infants and children up to 1 to 2 years)

$$\frac{\text{Age in months}}{150} \times \text{Adult dose} = \text{Infant's or child's dose}$$

CLARK'S RULE (for infants or children)

$$\frac{\text{Weight in pounds}}{150} \times \text{Adult dose} = \text{Infant's or child's dose}$$

Answers to Problems

When using the variable, yet acceptable, known equivalents, more than one correct answer is possible. Answers will vary according to the equivalent chosen for use. All answers should fall within the 10 percent margin of error allowed when doing the conversion. More than one answer is sometimes given; however, not all possible correct answers are included.

Intravenous flow rates can be approached in many ways. Not all possible ways are included.

Each answer or group of answers has the page number(s) in the text of the book to which the user can refer if the answer is incorrect.

CHAPTER 1 • Arithmetic Basics

Page 1

1. $\frac{1}{150}$ (see p. 5)
2. $\frac{3}{7}$ (see p. 5)
3. $\frac{100}{1}$ (see p. 5)
4. 0.03 (see p. 8)
5. 1:2 (see pp. 8 and 14)
6. $\frac{1}{5}\%$ (see pp. 8 and 11)

Page 2

7. $\frac{2}{100}$ (see p. 5)
8. 0.04 (see p. 8)
9. 0.066 (see p. 8)
10. $\frac{500}{150} = 3\frac{1}{3}$ (see pp. 5 and 6)
11. $\frac{17}{6} = 2\frac{5}{6}$ (see pp. 5 and 6)
12. $\frac{17}{12} = 1\frac{5}{12}$ (see pp. 5 and 6)
13. $\frac{2501}{1000}$ or $2\frac{501}{1000}$ (see pp. 5 and 6)

14. $^{20}\!/_{21}$ (see pp. 5 and 6)
15. $^{1}\!/_{50}$ (see pp. 5 and 6)
16. 2¼ (see pp. 5 and 6)
17. $2^{1}\!/_{12}$ (see pp. 5 and 6)
18. $^{7}\!/_{12}$% (see pp. 9 and 11)
19. 0.073 (see p. 9)
20. $^{13}\!/_{15}$ (see pp. 9 and 14)
21. 1½ (see p. 6)
22. $^{1}\!/_{300}$ (see p. 6)
23. ⅙ (see p. 6)
24. ⅙ (see p. 6)
25. 0.60 (see p. 9)
26. $^{1}\!/_{1000}$ (see pp. 6 and 7)
27. 0.06 (see pp. 9 and 10)
28. 500 (see pp. 6 and 7)
29. ⅓ (see pp. 6 and 7)
30. ½ (see pp. 6 and 7)
31. 4½ (see p. 7)
32. 1 (see p. 7)
33. 1⅛ (see p. 7)
34. 15 (see p. 10)
35. ⅔ or 0.67 (see pp. 7, 8, and 10)
36. ⅔ (see p. 7)
37. ¾ (see p. 7)
38. 0.1 (see pp. 7 and 8)
39. 0.02 (see p. 11)
40. 15.0 (see pp. 7 and 8)
41. 0.04 (see p. 14)
42. 3:100 (see p. 14)
43. 1:1 (see p. 15)
44. 75:100 or 3:4 (see pp. 4 and 14)
45. 1:1000 (see p. 14)
46. 5:1000 or 1:200 (see p. 15)
47. 125:100,000 = 1:800 (see p. 15)
48. ⅓% or 0.3% (see p. 11)
49. 50% (see p. 11)
50. $^{1}\!/_{10}$% or 0.1% (see p. 15)
51. 75% (see p. 11)
52. 250% (see p. 11)

Page 3

53. 2½ (see p. 13)
54. 20 (see p. 13)
55. 1½ (see p. 13)
56. 3200 (see p. 13)
57. 2½ (see p. 13)
58. 0.3 (see p. 9)
59. 0.7 (see p. 9)

60. 0.67 (see p. 9)
61. 0.33 (see p. 9)

For answers 62–71, see pp. 17 and 18

62. 9
63. 6
64. 90
65. 12
66. 60
67. iv
68. MM
69. vi
70. xv
71. C

For answers 72–81, see p. 15 and Figure 1–1

72. 36.11°C
73. −40°C
74. 43.33°C
75. 18.33°C
76. 40.56°C
77. 50°F
78. 104°F
79. 14°F
80. 89.6°F
81. 98.6°F

For answers 82–92, see pp. 18 and 19

82. 2430
83. 1620
84. 1015
85. 0730
86. 2100
87. 12 midnight
88. 12:15 AM
89. 9:00 PM
90. 3:30 PM
91. 9:00 AM
92. 7:30 AM

Page 19

For answers 1–5, see p. 5

1. ¾
2. ⅞
3. ¾
4. ⅓
5. ⅔

For answers 6–15, see pp. 5 and 6

6. $\frac{1}{100}$
7. $2\frac{1}{4}$
8. $2\frac{5}{6}$
9. $3\frac{5}{6}$
10. $1\frac{1}{1000}$
11. $2\frac{1}{2}$
12. $\frac{3}{200}$
13. $2\frac{7}{12}$
14. $2\frac{9}{20}$
15. $3\frac{1}{300}$

For answers 16–25, see p. 6

16. $\frac{1}{600}$

Page 20

17. $\frac{5}{6}$
18. $\frac{1}{4}$
19. $1\frac{2}{3}$
20. $\frac{1}{2000}$
21. $\frac{11}{12}$
22. $1\frac{1}{6}$
23. $66\frac{2}{3}$
24. $333\frac{1}{3}$
25. $\frac{2}{3}$

For answers 26–50, see pp. 6 and 7

26. $\frac{1}{6}$
27. $1\frac{7}{8}$
28. $3\frac{1}{2}$
29. $\frac{1}{500}$
26. $\frac{1}{8,000,000}$
31. $\frac{1}{100}$
32. $\frac{1}{12,000}$
33. $\frac{5}{32}$
34. 60
35. 1500
36. $\frac{1}{120}$
37. 8
38. 90
39. 96
40. $\frac{1}{10}$
41. $3\frac{3}{4}$
42. 4
43. 20,000
44. $\frac{1}{8}x$
45. 1x or x
46. $\frac{1}{100}$

47. $\frac{1}{200}$x
48. 21$\frac{1}{3}$
49. 20
50. 150

For answers 51–75, see p. 7

51. $\frac{8}{9}$
52. 1
53. 1$\frac{1}{2}$
54. 1
55. $\frac{3}{4}$
56. $\frac{15}{28}$
57. 3000
58. 666$\frac{2}{3}$
59. $\frac{1}{10}$
60. 1500
61. $\frac{5}{8}$
62. $\frac{1}{2}$

Page 21

63. 100
64. $\frac{3}{4}$
65. $\frac{3}{4}$
66. $\frac{1}{12}$
67. $\frac{1}{2}$
68. 111$\frac{1}{9}$
69. 240
70. 256
71. $\frac{1}{2}$
72. 85$\frac{1}{3}$
73. 80
74. $\frac{1}{75}$
75. $\frac{5}{6}$

For answers 76–85, see p. 5

76. $\frac{1}{3}$
77. $\frac{1}{200}$
78. $\frac{1}{10,000}$
79. $\frac{1}{300}$
80. $\frac{1}{300}$
81. $\frac{2}{4}$
82. $\frac{1}{2}$
83. $\frac{500}{1}$
84. $\frac{1}{64}$
85. $\frac{4}{3}$

For answers 86–95, see p. 5

86. 3.019
87. 0.002

88. 4.005
89. 60.40
90. 100.67
91. 64.35
92. 7.5
93. 1.15
94. 0.200
95. 0.0025

For answers 96–115, see pp. 7 and 8

96. 0.5
97. 0.005
98. 0.05
99. 0.01
100. 0.02
101. 0.75
102. 0.6⅔
103. 0.0001
104. 0.125
105. 2.25
106. 1/10,000

Page 22

107. 3/100
108. ½
109. 1/100
110. 1/200
111. ½
112. 27/100
113. 3/5
114. 1⅛
115. ¼

For answers 116–125, see p. 9

116. 4.0
117. 0.1
118. 6.0
119. 5.5
120. 0.1
121. 2.01
122. 5.01
123. 0.10
124. 1.00
125. 0.03

For answers 126–135, see p. 9

126. 0.01
127. 0.75
128. 0.55
129. 0.0036

130. 1.38
131. 0.056
132. 0.25
133. 0.0035
134. 0.125
135. 0.003

For answers 136–140, see pp. 9 and 10

136. 0.9375
137. 0.25
138. 0.001
139. 0.008
140. 0.0015

For answers 141–145, see p. 10

141. 0.01⅔
142. 20
143. 10
144. 1
145. 20

For answers 146–165, see pp. 10 and 11

146. 1/500
147. 1/1000
148. 3/20

Page 23

149. 1/1
150. 1/10,000
151. 12.5%
152. 0.01%
153. 150%
154. 1%
155. 0.2%
156. 0.001
157. 0.02
158. 0.5
159. 0.000125
160. 1.0
161. 0.4%
162. 333%
163. 90%
164. 1%
165. 667%

For answers 166–175, see p. 14

166. 1:60
167. 1000:1
168. 5:3
169. 5:10,000

170. 7:4
171. $\frac{1}{1000}$
172. $\frac{5}{100} = \frac{1}{20}$
173. $\dfrac{\frac{4}{10}}{1000} = \dfrac{4}{10,000} = \dfrac{1}{2500}$
174. $\dfrac{1}{1\frac{1}{2}} = \dfrac{2}{3}$
175. $\frac{100}{5} = 20$

For answers 176–185, see p. 14

176. 25:100 = 1:4
177. 0.1:100 = 1:1000
178. 550:100 = 5.5:1; 55:10 = 11:2
179. 80:100 = 4:5
180. 5:100 = 1:20
181. 0.0001
182. 0.005
183. 1.111
184. 100
185. 100,000

For answers 186–195, see p. 15

186. 0.9:100
187. 0.5:100 = 1:200

Page 24

188. 10:100 = 1:10
189. 3:100
190. 100:100 = 1:1
191. 2000%
192. 2%
193. 1.7%
194. 5%
195. 100,000%

For answers 196–215, see p. 13

196. 3
197. 20
198. 200,000
199. 6.4
200. 120
201. 8
202. 1⅔
203. 10
204. 2
205. 666⅔
206. 62½
207. 90
208. ¼

209. 5
210. 300,000
211. 3⅗
212. 8
213. 10
214. 1⅔
215. ¾

For answers 216–225, see pp. 15 and 16

216. 100°C
217. 0°C
218. 27.78°C
219. −17.78°C
220. 15.56°C
221. 32°F
222. 212°F
223. 68°F
224. 95°F
225. 104°F

For answers 226–235, see pp. 17 and 18

226. 19
227. 7
228. 90
229. 16
230. 60

Page 25

231. $\overline{\text{iv}}$
232. $\overline{\text{xii}}$
233. $\overline{\text{viii}}$
234. M
235. CL

For answers 236–245, see pp. 18 and 19

236. 1200
237. 0145
238. 1515
239. 2430
240. 1410
241. 12:00 midnight
242. 3:20 AM
243. 6:10 PM
244. 4:50 PM
245. 11:00 AM
   1. ¹⁄₁₅₀ (see p. 5)
   2. 0.5% (see pp. 7 and 8)
   3. ⅛₀₀₀ (see p. 5)
   4. 0.03 (see p. 8)

5. 0.5 (see p. 8)
6. $^{2}/_{1000}$ (see p. 5)

For answers 7–10, see p. 8

7. 1.266
8. 10.745
9. 5.0245
10. 2.60
11. $^{125}/_{10,000} = ^{1}/_{80}$ (see pp. 7 and 8)
12. $^{4}/_{1000} = ^{1}/_{250}$ (see pp. 10 and 11)
13. $^{1}/_{10,000}$ (see p. 14)
14. 0.08 (see p. 10)
15. 0.01 (see p. 14)
16. 0.04 (see pp. 7 and 8)
17. 2.5:1 or 5:2 (see p. 14)
18. 1:10,000 (see p. 14)
19. 2:1000 or 1:500 (see p. 15)

Page 26

20. 12.5% (see pp. 10 and 11)
21. 0.6$^{2}/_{3}$ % (see p. 11)
22. 0.01% (see p. 15)
23. 0.333 (see p. 9)
24. 0.667 (see p. 9)
25. 1.333 (see p. 9)
26. $^{1}/_{100}$ (see pp. 5 and 6)
27. 2$^{1}/_{6}$ (see pp. 5 and 6)
28. 0.000025 (see p. 10)
29. 0.5 (see p. 10)
30. $^{5}/_{6}$ (see p. 7)
31. 2,000 (see p. 7)
32. 1$^{1}/_{2}$ (see p. 6 and 7)
33. 1$^{2}/_{3}$ (see p. 10)
34. 200 (see p. 10)
35. 3 (see p. 7)
36. 1.95 (see p. 9)
37. $^{7}/_{80}$ or 0.0875 (see pp. 7 and 8, 9, 6 and 7)
38. $^{2}/_{3}$ (see p. 7)
39. 20 (see pp. 6 and 7)
40. 499$^{2}/_{3}$ (see p. 6)
41. 6 (see p. 10)
42. 333$^{1}/_{3}$ (see p. 6)
43. 50 (see pp. 9 and 10)
44. $^{1}/_{400}$ (see pp. 7 and 8, 9, 6 and 7)
45. 1$^{7}/_{12}$ (see pp. 5 and 6)
46. 0.000005 (see p. 10)
47. $^{1}/_{300}$ (see p. 6)
48. $^{1}/_{20}$ (see pp. 6 and 7)
49. 4$^{5}/_{12}$ (see pp. 5 and 6)

50. 1⅚ (see p. 6)
51. 2¹⁹⁄₂₀ (see p. 6)
52. 4 (see pp. 6 and 7)
53. 1⅞ (see p. 6 and 7)
54. 240 (see p. 7)

For answers 55–60, see p. 9

55. 0.1
56. 1.3
57. 4.5
58. 0.67
59. 1.00
60. 5.01

For answers 61–70, see p. 13

61. 7.5
62. 0.000025
63. 6

Page 27

64. ⁸⁄₁₅ or 0.53
65. 10
66. 20
67. 2000
68. **5**
69. 500
70. 0.5

For answers 71–90, see pp. 17 and 18

71. 4
72. 1½
73. 12
74. 2
75. 1000
76. 30
77. 15
78. 7½
79. 120
80. 15
81. īss
82. xxx
83. M
84. v̄īīss
85. xv
86. XC
87. iv
88. LX
89. CD
90. MMD

For answers 91–100, see pp. 15 and 16

91. 37°C
92. 93.3°C
93. −45.56°C
94. −12.2°C
95. 20°C
96. 100.4°F
97. 109.4°F
98. 50°F
99. 93.2°F
100. 14°F

For answers 101–110, see p. 18

101. 2430
102. 1620
103. 1015
104. 0730
105. 2100
106. 12 midnight

Page 28

107. 8:00 AM
108. 9:00 PM
109. 3:30 PM
110. 9:10 PM

1. $\frac{1}{150}$ is twice as large as $\frac{1}{300}$ (see p. 5)
2. $\frac{2}{3} + \frac{1}{4} = \frac{8}{12} + \frac{3}{12} = \frac{11}{12}$ (see pp. 5 and 6)
3. 0.01 (see pp. 7 and 8)
4. $125:100,000 = 1:800$ (see p. 15)
5. $1:1000 = 0.1:100 = 0.1\%$ (see p. 15)
6. 0.7 (see p. 9)
7. $60:1 = x:0.5;\ 1x = 60 \times 0.5;\ x = 30$ (see p. 13)
8. $(98 - 32)\dfrac{5}{9} = 66 \times \dfrac{5}{9} = \dfrac{330}{9} = 36.7°C$ (see p. 15)
9. 9 (see pp. 17 and 18)
10. $1\frac{1}{2} \div \frac{1}{2} = \frac{3}{2} \times \frac{2}{1} = \frac{6}{2} = 3$ (see p. 7)
11. $\frac{1}{60} \times 4 = \frac{1}{60} \times \frac{4}{1} = \frac{4}{60} = \frac{1}{15}$ (see p. 6 and 7)
12. 0.006 is $\frac{1}{5}$ of 0.03 (see p. 8)
13. $3:100$ (see p. 15)
14. $2x = \dfrac{300}{150};\ x = \dfrac{300}{150} \div \dfrac{2}{1};\ x = \dfrac{300}{150} \times \dfrac{1}{2};\ x = \dfrac{300}{300} = 1$ (see p. 13)
15. $(9 \times \frac{9}{5}) + 32 = \dfrac{81}{5} + 32 = 16.2 + 32 = 48.2°F$ (see p. 15)
16. $\overline{\text{viiss}}$ (see pp. 17 and 18)
17. $0.330 - 0.033 = 0.297$ (see p. 9)
18. $200,000:2 = 300,000:x;\ 200,000x = 600,000;\ x = \dfrac{600,000}{200,000} = 3$ (see p. 13)
19. $8\frac{1}{3} \times 15 = \frac{25}{3} \times \frac{15}{1} = \frac{25}{1} \times \frac{5}{1} = 125$ (see pp. 6 and 7)

20. $\dfrac{7.5}{100} = 0.075$ (see pp. 10 and 11)

21. $125:5 = 0.25:x$; $125x = 0.25 \times 5$; $125x = 1.25$; $x = 1.25 \div 125$; $x = 0.01$ (see p. 13)

22. $1:1000 = 0.005:x$; $1x = 1000 \times 0.005$; $x = 5$ (see p. 13)

23. $5\% = \dfrac{5}{100} = 0.05$ (see p. 10)

24. $0.25:5 = 0.3:x$; $0.25x = 1.5$; $x = 1.5 \div 0.25$; $x = 6$ (see p. 13)

25. $1500 \div 4 = \dfrac{1500}{1} \times \dfrac{1}{4} = \dfrac{1500}{4} = 375$ (see p. 7)

26. $\dfrac{1}{64}:1 = x:32$; $1x = \dfrac{1}{64} \times \dfrac{32}{1}$; $x = \dfrac{32}{64}$; $x = \dfrac{1}{2}$ (see p. 13)

27. $0.667 \times 100 = 66.7\%$ (see pp. 10 and 11)

28. $\dfrac{0.3 \times 500}{1.7} = \dfrac{150}{1.7} = 88.24$ (see p. 10)

29. $\dfrac{8}{8+12} \times 500 = \dfrac{8}{20} \times \dfrac{500}{1} = \dfrac{8}{1} \times \dfrac{25}{1} = 200$ or

$\dfrac{8}{20} \times \dfrac{500}{1} = \dfrac{2}{5} \times \dfrac{500}{1} = \dfrac{2}{1} \times \dfrac{100}{1} = 200$ (see pp. 6 and 7)

30. $1:64 = 1\dfrac{1}{2}:x$; $1x = \dfrac{64}{1} \times \dfrac{3}{2}$; $x = \dfrac{32}{1} \times \dfrac{3}{1}$; $x = 96$ (see p. 13)

31. $\frac{1}{10}\%$ is twice as large as $\frac{1}{20}\%$ (0.0010 versus 0.0005) (see p. 8)

32. $50:100$ or $1:2$ (see p. 15)

33. $1:15 = 8\dfrac{1}{3}:x$; $1x = \dfrac{15}{1} \times \dfrac{25}{3}$; $x = \dfrac{375}{3}$; $x = 125$ (see p. 13)

34. $0.5:100$ or $5:1000$ or $1:200$ (see p. 15)

35. $\dfrac{300}{24} \div 24 = \dfrac{3000}{1} \times \dfrac{1}{24} = \dfrac{3000}{24} = 125$ (see p. 7)

36. 0.67 (see p. 9)

37. $\dfrac{1}{60}:1 = x:2$; $1x = \dfrac{1}{60} \times \dfrac{2}{1}$; $x = \dfrac{2}{60}$; $x = \dfrac{1}{30}$ (see p. 13)

Page 29

38. $\frac{1}{120}$ is larger than $\frac{1}{150}$; $\frac{1}{150}$ is larger than $\frac{1}{200}$ (see p. 5)

39. $2 \div 100 = 0.002$ (see p. 14)

40. $4:1 = x:2$; $1x = 8$ (see p. 13)

41. $1:1000$ is one-tenth of $1:100$ (see pp. 5 and 14)

42. $0.25:1 = 0.5:x$; $0.25x = 0.5$; $x = 0.5 \div 0.25$; $x = 2$. (see p. 13)

43. $15:1 = x:0.3$; $1x = 15 \times 0.3$; $x = 4.5$. (see p. 13)

44. $1:100$ is 10 times as large as $1:1000$ (see pp. 5 and 14)

45. $\frac{1}{150} = 1 \div 150 = 0.006\frac{2}{3} = 0.7\%$ (see pp. 10 and 11)

46. $0.01:1 = x:5$; $1x = 0.01 \times 5$; $x = 0.05$. (see p. 13)

47. $2.2:1 = 18:x$; $2.2x = 18$; $x = 18 \div 2.2$; $x = 8.18$ (see p. 13)

48. $\dfrac{0.44 \times 0.5}{1.7} = \dfrac{0.22}{1.7} = 0.129$ (see p. 10)

49. $80:1 = x:1.3$; $1x = 1.3 \times 80$; $x = 104$. (see p. 13)

50. $100:16 = 40:x$; $100x = 40 \times 16$; $100x = 640$; $x = 6.4$ (see p. 13)

51. 12:00 midnight (see p. 18)

52. 2200 (see p. 18)

53. 8:10 PM (see p. 18)
54. 1600 (see p. 18)
55. 1:00 PM (see p. 18)
56. $^1/_{150}$ (see p. 5)
57. $^{10}/_{1000} + ^2/_{1000} = ^{12}/_{1000}$ or 0.012 (see pp. 5 and 6)
58. $^3/_2 - ^4/_3 = ^9/_6 - ^8/_6 = ^1/_6$ (see p. 6)
59. $^5/_2 - ^6/_5 = ^{25}/_{10} - ^{12}/_{10} = ^{13}/_{10} = 1^3/_{10}$ (see p. 6)
60. $^{19}/_3 - ^1/_6 = ^{38}/_6 - ^1/_6 = ^{37}/_6 = 6^1/_6$ (see p. 6)
61. $^{60}/_4 \times ^{15}/_1 = ^{900}/_4 = 225$ (see pp. 6 and 7)
62. $^{64}/_2 \div ^{16}/_2 = ^{64}/_2 \times ^2/_{16} = ^{128}/_{32} = 4$ (see p. 7)
63. $^{25}/_{1000} = ^1/_{40}$ (see pp. 7 and 8)
64. 0.7 (see p. 8)
65. 0.66 (see p. 8)
66. $^2/_{1000} = ^1/_{500}$ (see pp. 10 and 11)
67. 0.01:100 or 1:10,000 (see p. 15)
68. $^{1125}/_{1000} = 45:40 = 9:8$ (see p. 14)
69. 10 (see pp. 9 and 10)
70. 57.5 (see p. 10)

CHAPTER 2 • Overview

Page 44

For answers 1–50, see p. 36, Table 2–5, and pp. 39–44

1. 50 mg (15 gr:1000 mg); 45 mg (1 gr:60 mg); 48 mg (1 gr:64 mg); 48.75 mg (1 gr:65 mg)
2. 5 gr (1 gr:60 mg = x gr:300 mg [0.3 g]); 4½ gr (1 g:15 gr); 4⅘ gr (1 g:16 gr)

Page 45

3. 600 mg (1 g:1000 mg)
4. $^1/_{300}$ gr (1 gr:60 mg); $^3/_{1000}$ gr (15 gr:1000 mg)
5. 0.75 g (1000 mg:1 g)
6. 0.3 mg (1 gr = 60 mg); 0.33 mg (15 gr = 1g)
7. 0.5 g (15 gr:1 g)

Page 46

8. 8 mL (1 fl dr:4 mL)
9. 0.1 g (15 gr:1 g)
10. 300 mg (1 gr:60 mg); 320 mg (1 gr:64 mg); 325 mg (1 gr:65 mg); 312.5 mg (16 gr:1000 mg); 333.33 mg (15 gr:1000 mg)
11. 15 mL (1 tsp = 5 mL; 3 tsp = 1 Tbsp)
12. 30 mg (1 g:1000 mg)

Page 47

13. 59.09 or 59.1 kg (1 kg:2.2 lb)
14. 10 mL (1 tsp:5 mL)
15. 8 mL (8 fl dr:30–32 mL)
16. 5 fl dr (1 fl dr:4 mL)
17. $1\frac{2}{3}$ gr (1 gr = 60 mg); $1\frac{1}{2}$ gr

Page 48

18. 0.6, 0.66, or 0.67 g
19. 0.4 or 0.43 mg
20. 500 mg
21. $\frac{1}{6000}$ gr (1 gr = 60 mg); $\frac{1}{6666}$ gr (15 gr = 1 g)
22. 1 mg

Page 49

23. $\frac{5}{6}$ (1 gr = 60 mg); $\frac{3}{4}$ gr (15 gr = 1 g)
24. $\frac{1}{60}$, $\frac{1}{64}$, or $\frac{1}{65}$ gr
25. 0.3 mg
26. $1\frac{1}{2}$ gr
27. 5 gr (1 gr = 60 mg); 4.5 gr (15 gr = 1 g)

Page 50

28. 0.3 or 0.33 g
29. $\frac{1}{1500}$ or 0.00067 or 0.007 g
30. 300 mg
31. 3.75 fl dr (4 mL = 1 fl dr); 3 fl dr (5 mL = 1 fl dr)
32. 1500 mg

Page 51

33. 30 or 32 mL
34. 10 mg
35. $1\frac{1}{3}$ Tbsp (1 gr = 60 mg); $1\frac{1}{4}$ Tbsp (15 gr = 1 g)
36. 0.5 g
37. 13.2 lb

Page 52

38. 5 mg
39. 375 mL
30. 0.15 g
41. 3.18 kg
42. 83 mL
43. 121 lb

Page 53

44. 3 tsp
45. 81.8 kg
46. 11 lb
47. 2.5 kg

Page 54

48. 3.96 lb
49. 1.35 kg
50. 360 or 384 mL

CHAPTER 3 • Nonparenteral Drugs

Page 60

1. 1 tablet (see pp. 57 and 58, no. 3, and p. 59, no. 5)
2. 2 tablets (see pp. 59 and 60, no. 6)
3. 2 tablets of each drug (see p. 56, no. 1, and pp. 59 and 60, no. 6)

Page 61

4. ½ tablet (see p. 56, no. 1)
5. 2 tablets (see pp. 59 and 60, no. 6)

Page 62

6. 1 capsule (see p. 59, no. 5)
7. 2 tablets (see pp. 59 and 60, no. 6)
8. 1½ tablets (see p. 56, no. 1)

Page 63

9. 1 tablet (see pp. 59 and 60, no. 6)
10. 1 capsule (see pp. 56 and 57, no. 2)
11. 2 tablets (see pp. 59 and 60, no. 6)

Page 64

12. 1 tablet (see p. 59, no. 5)
13. 3 tablets (see p. 56, no. 1)
14. 4 tablets (see p. 56, no. 1)

Page 65

15. 2 tablets (see p. 56, no. 5)
16. 2 tablets (1 gr = 65 mg) (see pp. 57 and 58, no. 3)
17. 2 tablets (see p. 56, no. 1)

Page 66

18. 1 capsule (see p. 59, no. 5)
19. 1 tablet (see pp. 59 and 60, no. 6)
20. 1 tablet (see pp. 59 and 60, no. 6)
21. 2 tablets (see pp. 59 and 60, no. 6)

Page 67

22. 1 tablet (see pp. 59 and 60, no. 6)
23. ½ tablet (see pp. 59 and 60, no. 6)
24. 1 tablet (see pp. 59 and 60, no. 6)

Page 74

1. 4 mL (see pp. 68 and 69)

Page 75

2. 20 mL (see p. 71, no. 1)
3. 4 mL (see pp. 71 and 72, no. 2)
4. 5 mL (see p. 74, no. 6)

Page 76

5. 3.75 mL (see pp. 73 and 74, no. 5)
6. 10 mL (see pp. 68 and 69 and 73 and 74, no. 5)

Page 77

7. 7.5 mL (see pp. 73 and 74, no. 5)
8. 8 mL (see pp. 73 and 74, no. 5)
9. 4 mL (see p. 71, no. 1)

Page 78

10. 5 mL (see p. 36, Table 2–5, and p. 71, no. 1)
11. 20 mL, then 4 mL (see p. 71, no. 1)

Page 79

12. 9 mL (see pp. 73 and 74, Problem 5)
13. 8 (8.33) mL (see pp. 73 and 74, no. 5)
14. 7.5 mL (see pp. 73 and 74, no. 5)

Page 80

15. 20 mL (see pp. 73 and 74, no. 5)
16. 20 mL (see p. 71, no. 1)

Page 81

17. 4 mL (see pp. 71 and 72, no. 2, and p. 73, no. 4)
18. 27 mL (see pp. 73 and 74, no. 5)

Page 82

19. 15 mL (see p. 73, no. 4)
20. 1 mL (see p. 73, no. 4)

Page 88

1. 2 tsp in 1 qt (see pp. 85 and 86, no. 4)
2. 60 mL or 2 oz in 2 qt (see p. 85, no. 3)
3. 50 mL in 1 qt (see p. 85, no. 3)

Page 89

4. 2 mL in 100 mL (see pp. 84 and 85, no. 2)
5. 714$\frac{2}{7}$ mL alcohol and 1285$\frac{5}{7}$ mL water (see p. 85, no. 3)
6. 2 oz 5% dextrose in 2 oz water (see p. 85, no. 3)

Page 90

7. 10 mL 3% hydrogen peroxide and 20 mL water (see pp. 84 and 85, no. 2)
8. 1666$\frac{2}{3}$ mL 70% alcohol and 333$\frac{1}{3}$ mL water (see pp. 84 and 85, no. 2, and p. 85, no. 3)
9. 200 mL 5% sodium hypochlorite and 1800 mL sterile water (see p. 85, no. 3)

Page 91

10. 200 mL 5% boric acid and 300 mL sterile water (see p. 85, no. 3)

CHAPTER 4 • Parenteral Drugs

Page 97

1. 1 mL (see p. 96, no. 4)
2. 0.8 mL (see p. 96, no. 4)

Page 98

3. 1.33 mL (see p. 96, no. 4)
4. 2 mL (see p. 96, no. 4)

Page 99

5. 2 mL (see p. 96, no. 4)
6. 0.125 mL (see p. 96, no. 4)
7. 0.8 mL (see p. 96, no. 4)

Page 100

8. 0.5 mL (see p. 96, no. 4)
9. 0.2 mL (see pp. 95 and 96, no. 3)

Page 101

10. 2 mL, then 1 mL as needed for nausea (see pp. 94 and 95, no. 1)
11. 1.5 mL (see p. 96, no. 4)
12. 1.5 mL (see p. 96, no. 4)

Page 102

13. 2 mL (see p. 96, no. 4)

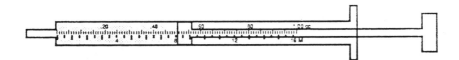

14. 0.5 mL or 8 m (see p. 96, no. 4)

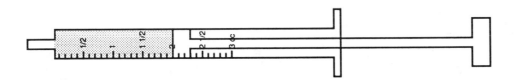

15. 0.4 mL or 6.4 m (see p. 96, no. 4)

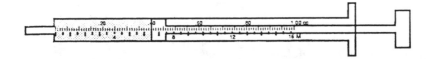

Page 103

16. 1 mL (see p. 96, no. 4)

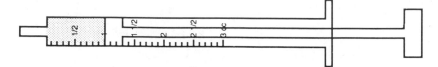

17. 2 mL (see p. 96, no. 4)

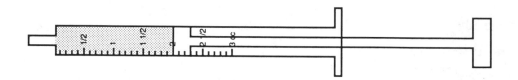

18. 0.5 mL (see p. 96, no. 4)

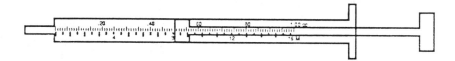

Page 104

19. 1.5 mL (see pp. 94–95, no. 1)

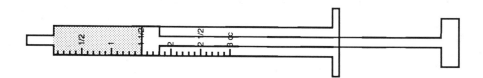

20. 2 mL (see p. 96, no. 4)

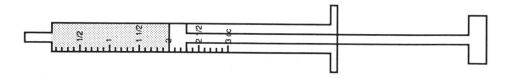

Page 112

1. 4 mL diluent, 5 mL drug (see p. 112, no. 6)

Page 113

2. 3.5 mL diluent, 2 mL drug (see pp. 111 and 112, no. 5)
3. 3 mL diluent, 1.67 mL drug (see p. 112, no. 6)

Page 114

4. 3 mL diluent, 2.5 mL drug (see p. 112, no. 6)
5. 1.4 mL diluent, 1.5 mL drug (see pp. 111 and 112, no. 5)
6. 2 mL diluent, 2 mL drug (see p. 112, no. 6)

Page 115

7. 1.8 mL diluent, 1 mL drug (see pp. 110–111, no. 3)
8. 3.2 mL diluent, 2.67 mL drug (see p. 112, no. 6)

Page 116

9. 3.2 mL diluent, 1 mL drug (see p. 109, no. 1)
10. 8.6 mL diluent, 2 mL drug (see p. 112, no. 6)

Page 117

11. 4 mL diluent, 5 mL drug (see p. 112, no. 6)
12. 2.5 mL diluent, 3 mL drug (see p. 112, no. 6)

Page 118

13. 2 mL of diluent to 1 g vial, 1.5 mL drug (see p. 111, no. 4)

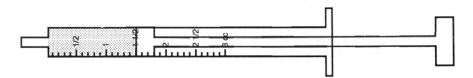

14. 12 mL of diluent, 2 (2.08) mL drug (see pp. 111 and 112, no. 5)

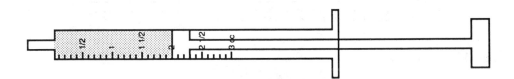

Page 119

15. 3.5 mL of diluent, 3 mL drug (see pp. 111 and 112, no. 5)

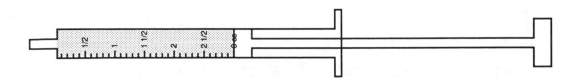

Page 120

16. 3 mL of diluent, 2.6 mL drug (see p. 112, no. 6)

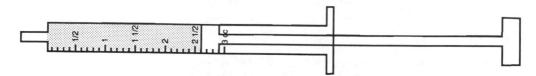

17. 1.4 mL of diluent to each of two 250 mg vials, total resulting volume of each vial (see pp. 111 and 112, no. 5)

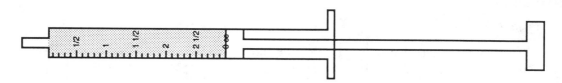

Page 121

18. 2 mL of diluent, 1.0 mL drug (see p. 112, no. 6)

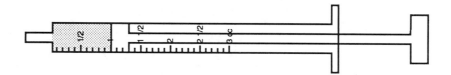

19. 4 mL of diluent to 1,000,000 U vial, 0.5 mL drug (see pp. 110 and 111, no. 3)

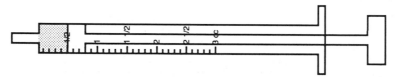

Page 122

20. 8.6 mL of diluent, 1.2 mL drug (see pp. 111 and 112, no. 5)

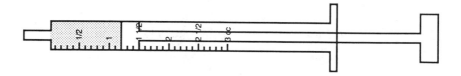

Page 130

1. 0.1 mL drug in tuberculin syringe (see p. 128, no. 1)
2. 0.18 mL drug in tuberculin syringe (see p. 128, no. 1)
3. 0.95 mL drug (see p. 129, no. 2, and pp. 129 and 130, no. 3)

Page 131

 4. Novalin R to 24 U mark, then Novalin N to 69 U mark (see p. 125, first paragraph)
 5. 88 U (see p. 128, no. 1)

Page 132

 6. 37 U (see p. 125, first paragraph)
 7. 92 U (see p. 125, first paragraph)
 8. 17 U (see p. 125, first paragraph)
 9. 24 U (see p. 125, first paragraph)

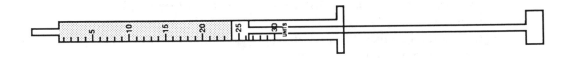

10. Novalin R to 15 U mark and Novalin L to the 45 U mark (see p. 125, first paragraph)

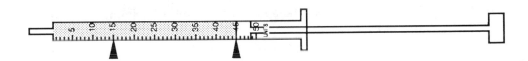

11. 0.75 mL (see p. 128, no. 1)

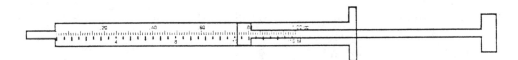

12. 83 U (see p. 125, first paragraph)

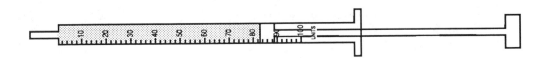

Page 136

 1. 42 gtts/min (see p. 135)

Page 137

 2. 62 or 63 gtts/min (see p. 134)
 3. 14 gtts/min (see p. 135)

4. 42 gtts/min (see p. 135)
5. Slow flow to 21 gtts/min in order to give each 1000 mL in 8 h. At 1800 h, regulate second bottle at 31 gtts/min (see p. 136, no. 3).

Page 138

6. Speed up flow to 44 gtts/min in order to give second 1000 mL in 8 h. (see p. 136, no. 3)
7. 17 gtts/min (see p. 136, no. 4)
8. 33 gtts/min (see p. 135)
9. 31 gtts/min (see p. 134)

Page 139

10. D-5-W at 33 gtts/min, then ⅙ Ringer's at 17 gtts/min (see p. 135)
11. 42 gtts/min (see p. 135)
12. 50 gtts/min for 1 h, then 12 or 13 gtts/min (see p. 134)
13. 31 gtts/min (see p. 134)

Page 140

14. 50 gtts/min initially; at 1830 h regulate at 43 gtts/min to give 1200 mL in 7 h (see p. 136, no. 3)
15. D-5-W at 55 or 56 gtts/min, then 0.45 NaCl at 17 gtts/min. At 1400 reset the 0.45% NaCl to 10 gtts/min for the remaining 250 mL of solution to run over the next 4 h (see p. 136, no. 5).

Page 145

1. Use 10 mL diluent; put all of drug in 100 mL PB bag; and regulate 110 mL at 55 gtts/min (110 mL/½ h × 4 = 55 gtts/min) to give in 30 min (see pp. 143 and 144, no. 2).
2. Use 10 mL diluent; flush heparin lock with isotonic NaCl; give all of drug in 3–5 min into heparin lock; and flush heparin lock with isotonic NaCl then heparin (see pp. 141–143, and 144 and 145, no. 3).

Page 146

3. Withdraw 20 mL diluent from 100 mL IV bag; add 10 mL to each of two 500 mg vials of drug; add all of reconstituted drug back to 100 mL IV bag; and regulate PB at 20 gtts/min (100 mL/1 h × 6 = 17 gtts/min) to give in 1 h (see pp. 143 and 144, no. 2).

Page 147

4. Add ⅓ of dissolved drug to 50 mL (minimum of 10 mL and maximum of 100 mL) PB bag; flush heparin lock with isotonic NaCl; regulate PB at 25 gtts/min (50 mL/½ h × 4 = 25 gtts/min) for 30 min; and flush heparin lock with isotonic NaCl then heparin (see pp. 144 and 145, no. 3).
5. Add 3.2 mL diluent to drug vial; mix; add all 4 mL of the reconstituted drug to 50 mL IV fluid; flush heparin lock with isotonic NaCl; regulate IV flow between 25 gtts/min (to run 30 min) and 50 gtts/min (to run 15 min); and flush heparin lock with isotonic NaCl then heparin (see pp. 144 and 145, no. 3).

Page 148

6. Add 1.75 mL of drug to 50 mL bag of D-5-W and regulate flow between 4 gtts/min (to run 2 h) and 17 gtts/min (to run 30 min) (see pp. 143 and 144, no. 2).

7. Withdraw all 10 mL of drug; flush heparin lock with isotonic NaCl; give the drug over a 10 min period; and flush heparin lock with isotonic saline then heparin (see pp. 144 and 145, no. 3).

Page 149

8. Add 3.2 mL diluent to drug vial; add all 5 mL of reconstituted drug to 1000 mL of D-5-W IV fluid; and regulate flow at 21 gtts/min (see pp. 143 and 144, no. 2).

9. Give ½ mL (5000 U) heparin stat. Add 3 mL of heparin to 1000 mL of 0.45% sodium chloride IV solution, and invert bag at least six times to thoroughly mix the heparin into the solution; start IV; regulate flow at 7 gtts/min; and inject 0.5 mL of heparin into the flashball (see pp. 144 and 145, no. 3).

Page 150

10. Add 2 mL of drug to 50 mL D-5-W, and give PB at 33 gtts/min; 4 h later add 1 mL of drug to 50 mL D-5-W, and give PB at 17 gtts/min (see pp. 144 and 145, no. 3).

Page 154

1. Add 5.7 mL diluent; put 2 mL reconstituted drug in 50 mL (maximum of 100 mL, minimum of 33.3 mL) IV fluid in burette; regulate flow at 100 gtts/min (10 mL/min = 100 gtts/min); empty burette; and add 25 mL IV fluid (15 mL/h plus 10 mL reserve) to burette (see p. 153, no. 2).

2. Since 720 mL/24 h of IV fluid is ordered, use 1000 mL bag of IV fluid. Every 12 h put 0.25 mL of drug in burette and fill burette to 30 mL. Continue flow at 7.5 or 8 gtts/min. When burette is empty at end of hour, put 40 mL IV fluid in burette and continue flow at 8 gtts/min (see pp. 152 and 153, no. 1).

Page 155

3. If 0.5 g should be added to 100–200 mL IV fluid, then 100 mg should be added to 20–40 mL of IV fluid. Add 2 mL of drug to the end-of-hour 10 mL residual in the burette. Add 18 mL of the primary IV solution to the burette to a total of 30 mL, and continue flow at 30 gtts/min or 30 mL/h (see pp. 153 and 154, no. 3).

4. Dissolve drug in 10 mL of diluent; add all of reconstituted drug to 10 mL remaining in burette; add 80 mL D-5-W or fill burette to 100 mL mark; and regulate flow at 50 gtts/min to give in 30 min or at 75 gtts/min to give in 20 min. When burette is completely empty, add 15 mL of D-5-W (5 mL/h plus 10 mL residual) (see pp. 152 and 153, no. 1, and p. 153, no. 2).

Page 156

5. Add 3 mL (1.5 vials) of drug to 10 mL remaining in burette; fill burette with D-5-W to 100 mL mark; and continue flow at 100 mL/h or at 17 gtts/min. At end of 1 h, add 110 mL to empty burette (100 mL/h plus 10 mL reserve) (see pp. 152 and 153, no. 1, and p. 153, no. 2).

Page 162

1. Add 10 mL from 100 mL fluid bag to drug vial; dissolve drug; add entire amount of drug to the 100 mL IV bag; regulate flow at maximum of 300 mL/h (100 mL:20 min = x mL:60 min); or regulate at 100 mL/h to give in 1 h (see pp. 160 and 161, no. 5).
2. Add 20 mL of drug to 500 mL of D-5-W, and regulate to flow at 30 mL/h (see pp. 158 and 159, no. 2).

Page 163

3. Regulate flow at 120 mL/h (10,000 mcg [10 mg]:500 mL = 40 mcg/min:x mL/min) (see pp. 158 and 159, no. 2).
4. Put 3.125 mL of drug into 50 mL IV bag (5 mL:75 mL = 3.125 mL:x mL; x = 46.875 mL minimum fluid); regulate flow at 50–53 mL/h (see p. 158, no. 1).

Page 164

5. Add 10 mL (5 mEq) of drug to 50 mL bag of D-5-W (total of 60 mL [1 mEq:12 mL = 5 mEq:x mL]) and regulate flow at 12 mL/h (see pp. 158 and 159, no. 2).
6. Add 200 mg (5 mL) of drug to 250 mL D-5-W. To give 150 mcg/min, give 0.15 mg/min or 9 mg/h. To give 9 mg/h (200 mg:255 mL = 9 mg:x mL), set the volume delivery pump at 11.5 mL/h initially (see p. 159, no. 3).

Page 165

7. Add 1.75 mL of drug to 250 mL bag of D-5-W. Switch to PB rate of 200 mL/h for 1¼ h (200 mL:1 h = 250 mL:x h) to give drug at same rate as mL/h ordered. At end of 1¼ h, switch to primary rate of 200 mL/h (see p. 161, no. 6).
8. Add 0.8 mL of drug to 50 mL bag of D-5-W and run at 200 mL/h (50 mL:½ h = x mL:1 h) (see pp. 160 and 161, no. 5).

Page 166

9. Start IV with 50 mL bag of D-5-W and give 2.5 mL (55 lb = 25 kg; 0.01 mg:1 kg = x mg:25 kg; 1 mg:10 mL = 0.25 mg:x mL) of 1:10,000 epinephrine into flashball (see pp. 159 and 160, no. 4).
10. Give 2 mL of atropine (0.1 mg/mL) into flashball immediately. (44 lb = 20 kg; 0.01 mg:1 kg = x mg:20 kg; and 1 mg:10 mL = 0.2 mg:x mL) (see pp. 159 and 160, no. 4).

Page 169

1. Mix 25 U of insulin in 50 mL of IV fluid and regulate at 2 mL/h (see pp. 168 and 169, nos. 2 and 3).

Page 170

2. Mix 2 mL of heparin in total of 50 mL of IV fluid and regulate at 2 mL/h (see pp. 168 and 169, nos. 2 and 3).

3. Add 10 or 20 mL diluent as needed; withdraw all of drug (250,000 mcg); fill syringe to 50 mL; mix; and regulate at 3 mL/h (250 mcg : 1 min = x mcg : 60 min; 250,000 mcg : 50 mL = 15,000 mcg : x mL) (see pp. 168 and 169, no. 2).

Page 171

4. Reconstitute drug with 10 mL diluent; withdraw ½ of drug; add IV fluid to a total of 40 mL; and regulate at 40 mL/h (see p. 168, no. 1).

Page 172

5. To give 42 mcg/min or 2.52 mg/h, add 1.6 (1.575) mL or 63 mg of dopamine to a 50 mL bag of D-5-W. This is the amount of drug needed to run for 25 h. Set the auto syringe at 2 mL/h (see pp. 168 and 169, nos. 2 and 3).
6. Give 2 mL of heparin IV stat. In 4 h, add 1 mL of heparin to 50 mL bag of 0.9% NaCl; mix; withdraw all of the solution into a 60 mL syringe; and set the Harvard infuser to run at 100 mL/h. Follow heparin lock irrigation procedure (see p. 168, no. 1).
7. Add 1.9 (1.875) mL of gentamicin to a 50 mL bag of 0.9% NaCl; mix; withdraw all of the solution into a 60 mL syringe; and set syringe infuser to run at 25 mL/h. Follow heparin lock irrigation procedure (see p. 168, no. 1).

Page 173

8. Dissolve drug in 3–5 mL of sterile water; add ⅔ of the total amount of reconstituted drug to a 50 mL bag of D-5-W; withdraw all of the drug solution into a 60 mL Monoject syringe; and set syringe infuser to run at 50 mL/h. Follow heparin lock irrigation procedure (see p. 168, no. 1).

Page 177

For answers 1–8, see pp. 176 and 177

1. 75 kg; 2600 mL/day (Guide 2)

Page 178

2. 37.5 mL q3h (Guide 1)
3. 5 kg; 83.3 mL q4h (Guide 2)
4. 72.5 mL q4h (Guide 1)
5. 45.5 kg; 2010 mL/day (Guide 2)

Page 179

6. 150 mL q4h (Guide 1)
7. 1800 mL/day (Guide 1)
8. 10 kg; 41⅔ mL/h (Guide 2)

Page 181

For answers 1–8, see pp. 179–181

1. 340 calories
2. 170 calories

Page 182

3. 748 calories (170 from dextrose, 28 from amino acids, and 550 from fat emulsion)
4. 110 calories
5. 1648 calories (140 from amino acids, 1100 from fatty acids, and 408 from dextrose)
6. 790 calories (70 from amino acids, 550 from fatty acids, and 170 from dextrose)

Page 183

7. 210 calories
8. 1374 calories (1100 from lipids, 70 from amino acids, and 204 from dextrose)

CHAPTER 5 • Pediatric and Geriatric Dosages

Page 191

1. BSA = 0.87 m^2 (see p. 187, Fig. 5.1)
   The 100 mg tid ordered is less than the 127.94 mg tid recommended. Give 1 capsule (see p. 190, no. 3).
2. 17.5 lb = 8 kg (see p. 186)
   The 400 mg/day ordered is equal to the 400 mg maximum per day recommended. Give 0.4 mL of the reconstituted drug.

Page 192

3. BSA = 0.535 m^2, 26 lb = 11.8 kg
   The 225 mg/day ordered is less than the 236 mg/day recommended using the mg/kg/day guideline, and the 75 mg q8h ordered is less than the 78.7 mg q8h recommended using the adult dose guidelines. Give 3 mL q8h (see pp. 188 and 190, nos. 1 and 2).
4. 44 lb = 20 kg
   The 1000 mg/day ordered equals the 1000 mg minimum per day recommended. Give 0.65 mL of the reconstituted drug (see pp. 188 and 189, no. 1).

Page 193

5. BSA = 0.97 m^2
   The 50 mg/day ordered is considerably less than the 171.176 mg calculated. Give ½ scored tablet (see p. 190, no. 3).

6. BSA = 0.88 m²
   The 300 mg/day ordered is less than 396 mg maximum per day calculated. Give 0.67 mL of the drug (see pp. 188 and 189, no. 1, substituting m² for kg).

Page 194

7. 8 kg = 17.6 lb
   The 0.05 mg ordered is less than the maximum of 0.0704 mg preoperatively recommended. Give 0.25 mL of the drug (see pp. 188 and 189, no. 1, substituting lb for kg).

8. The 100 mcg/day ordered is much less than the 700 mcg/day recommended. Give 0.5 mL of the drug (see pp. 188 and 189, no. 1, substituting mcg for mg).

Page 195

9. The 50 mg q4h ordered is more than the 32 mg q3–4h maximum children's dose recommended, but it is equal to the lower adult dose. Give 1 tablet (see pp. 190 and 191, no. 4, substituting lb for kg).

Page 196

10. The 40 mg q8h ordered is a little less than the 44 mg q8h recommended. Give 0.8 mL of the drug (see pp. 190 and 191, no. 4).

11. The 60 mg/day ordered is less than 63.75 mg recommended (half way between the amount recommended for 4.0–4.5 kg of weight). Give 0.53 mL of the drug (see pp. 188 and 189, no. 1).

Page 197

12. 85 lb = 38.6 kg
    The 500 mg q6h ordered is slightly more than the 482.5 mg q6h recommended but it is within a 10% margin of error. Give 5 mL of the drug (see pp. 188 and 189, no. 1).

13. 40 lb = 18.18 kg, BSA = 0.75 m²
    The 0.2 mg ordered stat and q4h prn is slightly more than the 0.18 mg recommended using the mg/kg guideline, but it is less than the 0.225–0.375 mg recommended using the BSA guideline. Give 0.2 mL of the drug (see pp. 188 and 189, no. 1, substituting dose for day and substituting m² of BSA for kg).

Page 198

14. 22 lb = 10 kg, BSA = 0.465 m²
    The 15 mg q6h is slightly more than the 12.5 mg recommended using the mg/kg guideline, but it is less than the 17.44 mg recommended using the BSA guideline. Give 0.3 mL of the drug. (see pp. 188 and 189, no. 1, using mg/kg/day guideline and substituting m² for kg using BSA guideline).

15. 4000 g = 4 kg
    The 400 kg initial dose and the 300 mg q6h for 3 days are exactly the dosages recommended. Add 7.2 mL of diluent of the 1 g vial, mix, withdraw 1.6 mL of reconstituted drug, and add it to an appropriate amount of IV fluid for the initial

dose. For the 300 mg q6h doses, add 1.2 mL of the reconstituted drug to an appropriate amount of IV fluid (see pp. 190 and 191, no. 4).

Page 199

16. 9 lb = 4.1 kg
    The 10 mg q8h is slightly less than the 10.25 mg q8h calculated. Give 1.0 mL of the drug (see pp. 188 and 189, no. 1).
17. The 200,000 U q6h is within the range of 500,000–1,000,000 U/day recommended (200,000 U × 4 doses per day = 800,000 U/day). Add 4 mL of diluent to the 1,000,000 U vial, mix, and give 0.8 mL of the drug q6h (see pp. 189 and 190, no. 2).

CHAPTER 6 • Comprehensive Review Problems

Page 203

1. 10 gr (see p. 36, Table 2–5, and pp. 39–44)
2. 0.05 g (see p. 36, Table 2–5, and pp. 39–44)
3. 100 mg (15 gr:1000 mg); 90 mg (1 gr:60 mg); 96 mg (1 gr:64 mg); 97.5 mg (1 gr:65 mg) (see p. 36, Table 2–5, and pp. 39–44)

Page 204

4. ¾ gr (15 gr:1000 mg); ⅚ gr (1 gr:60 mg); ¹⁰⁄₁₃ gr (1 gr:65 mg) (see p. 36, Table 2–5, and pp. 39–44)
5. 0.6 mL (see p. 96, no. 4)
6. 21.08 or 21 gtts/min (see pp. 135 and 136)
7. 0.5 mL (see p. 128, no. 1)

Page 205

8. 2 tablets (see pp. 56 and 57, no. 2)
9. 0.4 mL (see p. 85, no. 3, and p. 69, last paragraph, and p. 70, first paragraph)
10. 357⅐ mL of 70% alcohol and 642⁶⁄₇ mL of water (see p. 87, no. 3)
11. 1 mL hydroxyzine hydrochloride and 0.75 mL meperidine hydrochloride (see p. 96, no. 4)

Page 206

12. 0.67 mL (see p. 96, no. 4)
13. 11.25 mL (see pp. 73 and 74, no. 5)
14. 4 tsp in 2000 mL of water (see pp. 85 and 86, no. 4)
15. 0.8 mL (see pp. 111 and 112, no. 5)

Page 207

16. 1 tablet (see pp. 56 and 57, no. 2)
17. 7.5 mL (see pp. 73 and 74, no. 5)
18. 0.3 mg or 3 mL (see p. 96, no. 4, and p. 59, no. 5)
19. 15 U mark with Novolin R then to 45 U mark with Novolin N (see p. 125, first paragraph, and p. 129, no. 2)

Page 208

20. 2 tablets (see pp. 56 and 57, no. 2)
21. Withdraw 0.05 mL of reconstituted drug into a tuberculin syringe; add diluent to a total of 1 mL; and administer at 2 mL/h with an auto syringe (see p. 168, no. 1).
22. Dissolve 1 tablet in 3 tsp of water and give 1 tsp (see pp. 83 and 84, no. 1, sol. 1).

Page 209

23. Using a 6 mL syringe, add 1 mL of diluent to the 125 mg vial to reconstitute the drug; withdraw 0.8 mL of reconstituted drug; add diluent to bring the volume up to 5 mL of drug in solution; and give into the proper IV portal at rate of 1 mL/min (see pp. 159 and 160, no. 4).
24. 10.9$^+$ kg (see p. 186)
    The 75 mg ordered is slightly more than the 72.67 mg maximum recommended but within the 10% margin of error. Give 3 mL of the drug (see pp. 188 and 189, no. 1).

Page 210

25. The ordered dose is almost equal to the 20.5 mg recommended. Give 0.8 mL of the drug (see pp. 188 and 189, no. 1).
26. Reconstitute the ampicillin as directed; add reconstituted drug to a 50 mL D-5-W PB bag; and infuse PB at rate of at least 8⅓ or 9 gtts/min in order to give the drug within 1 h. Add 2.67 mL clindamycin to a 50 mL (33.3 mL minimum of fluid) D-5-W PB bag; regulate to run a minimum of 33.3 min or at least 15 gtts/min. (These drugs are incompatible when mixed together so do not give one immediately after the other and be sure to flush the tubing with fluid from the ongoing IV before beginning the second drug administration (see pp. 135, 143, no. 1, and 144 and 145, no. 3).

Page 211

27. Expel all but 0.5 mL of the drug from the Tubex syringe and slowly give the 0.5 mL of the drug into the flashball while temporarily occluding the IV tubing above the injection site (see pp. 159 and 160, no. 4).
28. 25 gtts/min (see p. 136, no. 3)
29. 0.3 mL of Novolin L and then to 0.4 mL with Novolin R (see p. 125, first paragraph, and p. 129, no. 2)

Page 212

30. Add all of the reconstituted drug to the burette; fill the burette to 100 mL and continue to infuse at 24 mL/h since the drug should be given in a minimum of 2½ h (see pp. 152 and 153, no. 1).
31. 1 caplet (see pp. 56 and 57, no. 2)
32. 2 mL (see p. 96, no. 4)

Page 213

33. 200 mL 5% boric acid and 300 mL sterile water (see p. 85, no. 3)
34. 400 mL sodium bicarbonate in 2000 mL sterile water (see p. 85, no. 3)
35. 1 mg (see p. 36, Table 2–5, pp. 39–44)
36. 37.5 mL (see p. 176.)

Page 214

37. The 300 mg/day ordered is the maximum dose of 300 mg recommended. Give 0.5 mL of the drug. (see pp. 188 and 189, no. 1)
38. 10 mL (see p. 71, no. 1)
39. 21 gtts/min initially; at 1400 h regulate at 10 gtts/min (see p. 136, no. 5)

Page 215

40. 1000 mg (see p. 36, Table 2–5, and pp. 39–44)
41. 9 g (2 tsp) of salt in 1000 mL (1 qt) of water (see p. 84, no. 2)
42. 17 gtts/min (see pp. 134 and 135)
43. 84.375 mL (see p. 176)

Page 216

44. The 175 mg ordered is slightly less than the 180 mg recommended. Give 1.8 mL of the drug (see pp. 188 and 189, no. 1).
45. 5 mL (see pp. 68 and 69)
46. 42 gtts/min for 2 h then 21 gtts/min for 8 h (see p. 135)
47. 100 mcg (see p. 36, Table 2–5, and pp. 39–44)

Page 217

48. Add at least 10 mL diluent to 1 g vial; withdraw ¾ of drug solution; add IV fluid to a total of 50 mL; and regulate at 50 mL/h (see p. 168, no. 1).
49. 2918 mL (see p. 176)
50. Add 1.2 mL of diluent, withdraw 0.8 mL of drug solution, and add it to the 10 mL in burette at end of hour. Fill burette to 30 mL mark (minimum of 4.167 mL of fluid and maximum of 63.5 mL of solution) and continue flow at 30 gtts/min (30 mL/h). At end of hour when burette is empty, add 40 mL D-5-W (see p. 153, no. 2).

Page 218

51. 10 mcg (see p. 36, Table 2–5 and pp. 39–44)
52. ½ tablet (see pp. 59 and 60, no. 6)

53. 45.4 mL (see p. 176)
54. 0.9 mL of diluent to the 250 mg vial; 0.8 mL of drug (see p. 111, no. 4)
55. 3.4 mL of diluent to the 1 g vial; 3 mL of drug (see p. 111, no. 4)

Page 219

56. BSA = 0.75. The 8 mg ordered is a little less than the maximum of the range of 3.5–8.8 mg calculated. Give 1 mL of the drug (see p. 190, no. 3).
57. 1 mg (see p. 39, Table 2–5, and pp. 39–44)

Page 220

58. 1 mL (see p. 112, no. 6)
59. 25 gtts/min (see p. 135)
60. 274 calories (204 from dextrose and 70 from amino acids) (see pp. 180 and 181, no. 4)

Page 221

61. Add 3 mL diluent to vial, withdraw ½ of drug solution (about 1.5 mL), and add it to 10 mL in burette at end of hour. Fill burette with D-5-W to 50 mL mark and regulate flow at 50 gtts/min (50 mL/h). After the burette empties, add 35 mL D-5-W (25 mL for next hour and 10 mL reserve). Resume flow at 25 gtts/min (see pp. 152 and 153, no. 1).
62. Using 80 mg/100 mL PB bag of theophylline, regulate volume delivery pump at 125 mL/h (see pp. 160 and 161, no. 5).

Page 222

63. 1 mg (see p. 36, Table 2–5 and pp. 39–44)
64. 2370 calories (510 from dextrose, 210 from amino acids, and 1650 from fatty acids) (see pp. 180 and 181, nos. 3 and 4)
65. Add 2.3 mL of D-5-W to 50 mg vial of drug; then add 2 mL of drug solution to 250 mL of D-5-W and protect from light. Regulate volume delivery pump at 60 mL/h (1 mL/min) for 5 min, checking BP frequently, then regulate as indicated by BP (see p. 159, no. 3).

Page 223

66. The 30 mg ordered is between the 24.7–49.4 mg q4h calculated. Give 0.6 mL of the drug (see pp. 189 and 190, no. 2).
67. Add 200 mg (5 mL) of drug to 250 mL of D-5-W. To give 100 mcg/min, give 0.1 mg/min or 6 mg/h. To give 6 mg/h (200 mg : 255 mL = 6 mg : x mL), set pump at 7.6 or 7.7 mL/h initially (see p. 161, no. 6).
68. 1 mL (see pp. 94 and 95, no. 1)

Page 224

69. Mix 1.5 mL of heparin and 48.5 mL of IV fluid and regulate at 2 mL/h (see p. 169, no. 3).
70. 0.1 mL (see pp. 95 and 96, no. 3)
71. 510 calories (see p. 180, no. 1)

Page 225

72. 10 g (2 tsp) sugar to each 200 mL distilled water (see pp. 84 and 85, no. 2)
73. Mix 18.75 U of insulin in 50 mL of IV fluid and regulate at 2 mL/h (see pp. 168 and 169, no. 2)
74. 340 calories from D-10-W and D-5-W (see p. 180, no. 1)

Page 226

75. 1 mL (see p. 96, no. 4)
76. 8.6 mL diluent; 0.6 mL of drug (see pp. 111 and 112, no. 5)

Index

A page number followed by an ''f'' indicates a figure; a ''t'' following a page number indicates a table.

TABLE 2–6 • Abbreviations Used in Drug Administration

Abbreviation	Meaning	Abbreviation	Meaning
os	mouth	s̄	without
OU	both eyes	SC or sc	subcutaneously
oz	ounce	Sig or S	write on label
pc	after meals	sol	solution
per	by	sos	once if necessary
PO or per os	by mouth	sp	spirits
pm	when required	s̄s̄	a half
qh	every hour	stat	immediately
q2h	every 2 hours	supp	suppository
q3h	every 3 hours	syr	syrup
q4h	every 4 hours	tid	three times a day
qid	four times a day	tr or tinct	tincture
qod	every other day	U	unit
qoh	every other hour	ung	ointment
qs	quantity sufficient	vin	wine
Rx	take		

TABLE 2–5 • Most Frequently Used Approximate Equivalents

Fluid Units

Household	=	Metric	=	Apothecaries'
15 or 16 gtts		1 mL		15 or 16 m
2 Tbsp or 3 dssp or 6 tsp		30 or 32 mL		1 fl oz or 8 fl dr
2 glasses		500 mL		1 pt or 16 fl oz
4 glasses		1000 mL or 1 L		1 qt
		4000 mL		1 gal

STANDARD TIME	MILITARY TIME	STANDARD TIME	MILITARY TIME
12:01 AM	0001	12:00 noon	1200
12:15 AM	0015	12:30 PM	1230
1:00 AM	0100	1:00 PM	1300
1:30 AM	0130	2:00 PM	1400
2:00 AM	0200	3:00 PM	1500
3:00 AM	0300	4:00 PM	1600
4:00 AM	0400	5:00 PM	1700
5:00 AM	0500	6:00 PM	1800
6:00 AM	0600	7:00 PM	1900
7:00 AM	0700	8:00 PM	2000
7:30 AM	0730	8:30 PM	2030
8:00 AM	0800	9:00 PM	2100
9:00 AM	0900	10:00 PM	2200
9:45 AM	0945	11:00 PM	2300
10:00 AM	1000	11:03 PM	2303
11:00 AM	1100	12:00 midnight	2400

CALCULATION OF FLUID NEEDS
(see pp. 176–177 in text)
Guide 1: 1500 mL/m²/24 hours
Guide 2: a. 100 mL/kg for first 10 kg
    b. 50 mL/kg for next 10 kg
    c. 20 mL/kg for weight over 20 kg

CALCULATION OF CALORIES IN IV FLUIDS
(see pp. 179–181 in text)
Dextrose (Carbohydrate) = 3.4 calories/g
Amino-Acids (Protein) = 4 calories/g
Fatty Acids (Fats) = 11 calories/g

BODY SURFACE AREA FORMULA
(see pp. 187–188 in text)

$$\frac{\text{BSA in m}^2 \times \text{Adult dose}}{1.7} = \text{Infant's or child's dose}$$

TABLE 2–6 • Abbreviations Used in Drug Administration

Abbreviation	Meaning	Abbreviation	Meaning
āā	of each	H	by hypodermic
ac	before meals	h or hr	hour
ad lib	as desired	hs	hour of sleep
aq	water	IM	intramuscularly
aq dist or DW	distilled water	IV	intravenously
bid	twice a day	kg	kilogram
c̄	with	m	minim
caps	capsules	n, noc, or noct	night
comp	compound	non rep	not to be repeated
dil	dilute	NPO	nothing by mouth
elix	elixir	ol	oil
ext	extract	OD	right eye
fld or fl	fluid	od or qd	every day
g or Gm	gram	om or qam	every morning
gr	grain	on or qpm	every night
gtt	drop	OS	left eye

TABLE 2–5 • Most Frequently Used Approximate Equivalents

Weight Units

Household	=	Metric	=	Apothecaries'
		1 g or 1000 mg or 1,000,000 mcg		15–16 gr
		60, 64, or 65 mg		1 gr
2 Tbsp or 3 dssp or 6 tsp		30 or 32 g		1 oz or 8 dr
		1 kg or 1000 g		2.2 or 2.3 lb (imperial or avoirdupois, not apothecaries')

FORMULA A: EQUIVALENTS
(see pp. 39–44 and 56–60 in text)

KNOWN EQUIVALENTS	UNKNOWN EQUIVALENTS
(ORDERED)	(AVAILABLE)

$$15\ gr{:}1\ g = x\ gr{:}0.5\ g$$

or

$$1\ mL{:}16\ m = 0.5\ mL{:}x\ m$$

FORMULA B: PREPARING ORAL AND TOPICAL SOLUTIONS
(see pp. 83–87 in text)

KNOWN AMOUNTS	UNKNOWN AMOUNTS
(STRENGTH TO BE PREPARED)	(TOTAL TO BE PREPARED)

$$dosage{:}amount = dosage{:}amount$$
$$5\ g{:}100\ mL\ (5\%\ solution) = x\ g\ (mL){:}4000\ mL$$

Amount of drug needed using tablets, powders, or crystals:
$$1\text{–}30\ g{:}100\ mL = x\ g\ (of\ 70\%\ solution\ to\ make\ 30\%){:}2000\ mL$$
$$x = 600\ g\ needed$$

First and second steps of preparing weaker from stronger solutions:
$$2\text{–}70\ g{:}100\ mL = 600\ g{:}x\ mL\ (mL\ of\ 70\%\ solution)$$
$$x = 857\ mL\ needed$$

FORMULA B: DOSAGES
Dosages of tablets and oral or parenteral solutions:

KNOWN AMOUNTS	UNKNOWN AMOUNTS
(ORDERED)	(NEEDED)

$$dosage{:}amount = dosage{:}amount$$
$$5\ gr{:}1\ tablet = 15\ gr{:}x\ tablet(s)$$

or

$$250\ mg{:}1\ mL = 400\ mg{:}x\ mL$$

IV FLUIDS

CALCULATION OF DROPS PER MINUTE OR ML/H:
(see pp. 134–135 in text)

Macrodrip sets yielding 15 gtts/mL:
$$\frac{mL\ ordered}{h\ to\ run} \times 4 = gtts/min$$

Macrodrip sets yielding 10 gtts/mL:
$$\frac{mL\ ordered}{h\ to\ run} \times 6 = gtts/min$$

Microdrip sets yielding 60 gtts/mL:
$$\frac{mL\ ordered}{h\ to\ run} = mL/h = gtts/min$$

CALCULATION OF MAXIMUM STRENGTHS AND MINIMUM TIMES OF IV FLUIDS:
(see p. 144 in text)

Maximum strengths = Minimum IV fluid
$$12\ mg{:}1\ mL = 500\ mg\ (ordered){:}x\ mL$$

Maximum rate = Minimum time
$$30\ mg{:}1\ min = 500\ mg\ (ordered){:}x\ min$$